CELL BIOLOGY RESEARCH PROGRESS

ALKYLATING AGENTS AS ENVIRONMENTAL CARCINOGEN AND CHEMOTHERAPY AGENTS

CELL BIOLOGY RESEARCH PROGRESS

Additional books in this series can be found on Nova's website
under the Series tab.

Additional e-books in this series can be found on Nova's website
under the e-book tab.

CANCER ETIOLOGY, DIAGNOSIS AND TREATMENTS

Additional books in this series can be found on Nova's website
under the Series tab.

Additional e-books in this series can be found on Nova's website
under the e-book tab.

CELL BIOLOGY RESEARCH PROGRESS

ALKYLATING AGENTS AS ENVIRONMENTAL CARCINOGEN AND CHEMOTHERAPY AGENTS

YILDIZ DINCER
EDITOR

New York

For permission to use material from this book please contact us:
Telephone 631-231-7269; Fax 631-231-8175
Web Site: http://www.novapublishers.com

NOTICE TO THE READER

Library of Congress Cataloging-in-Publication Data

ISBN: 978-1-62618-487-9

Library of Congress Control Number: 2013935079

Published by Nova Science Publishers, Inc. † New York

Contents

Preface

Cancer is the second major cause of death in the world after cardiovascular diseases. Millions of people suffer from cancer not only in industrialized countries but also in developing countries. Although current improved techniques of cancer therapy increased the rate of recovery and survive a little bit, every year millions of people are diagnosed with cancer and more than half of the cancer patients die from it. Cancer is a disease that cells divide and grow uncontrollably forming malignant tumors which in turn, invade nearby organs. A tumor cell may also spread to distant organs through the lymphatic system or bloodstream, grow in new location and form a metastatic tumor there. Cancer is primarily an environmental disease with 90-95% of cases attributed to environmental factors and 5-10% due to genetic heritage. Environmental factors contributing cancer development include diet, obesity, tobacco, infections, radiation and chemical pollutants. Generally, majority of environmental factors are associated to life-style of individuals. It is nearly impossible to reveal what caused a cancer in any individual, because most cancers have multiple possible causes, and susceptibilities of individuals to cancer development are different. However it is fact that, in the presences of numerous risk factors cancer incidence increases. Although the role of lifestyle-related factors in cancer development is known, they are ignored generally. Alkylating agents, an important class of chemical carcinogens, is the most common environmental factor people exposed. Their precursors are present in vegetables, drinking water, beer, tobacco, various drugs, processed cheese, meat and fish products. Especially smoked, curred meats such as ham, sausage, bacon, salami which are frequently consumed are the major sources. Alkylating agents are also produced in stomach and gut, in vivo. Alkylating agents interact with DNA to form cytotoxic and mutagenic base adducts. O^6 methylguanine (O^6 MG) formed in cellular DNA by alkylating agents is a mutagenic lesion. O^6-MG adducts are repaired by the DNA repair protein, O^6-methylguanine DNA methyltransferase (O^6-MGMT). This enzyme repairs O^6-MG adducts by transferring the methyl group to itself at a specific cysteine residue and becomes inactivated. De novo synthesis of new enzyme molecules is required for subsequent repair activity. The susceptibility of a cell to alkylation damage is closely related to efficiency of repair by O^6-MGMT. Cells with low O^6-MGMT level are more susceptible to cytotoxic and mutagenic effects of alkylating agents. Because of their lethal effects, alkylating agents are used in certain chemotherapy protocols, and one of the major alternatives for the clinicians. Tumors resistant to conventional agents are disappeared by the action of alkylating agents. The presence of high levels of O^6-MGMT in tumors causes a powerful resistance to alkylating agent-based chemotherapy.

In the present book structure and carcinogenic mechanism of alkylating agents were reviewed. Their availability in frequently consumed foods were emphasized. Major classes of alkylating agents used in chemotherapy and usage of temozolomide, a new generation alkylating agent, in brain tumors were assessed. Primary goal of this book is to maintain awareness about alkylating agent exposure in modern life.

Yildiz Dincer

In: Alkylating Agents …
Editor: Yildiz Dincer

ISBN: 978-1-62618-487-9
© 2013 Nova Science Publishers, Inc.

Chapter I

Carcinogenesis

Yildiz Dincer[*]

Istanbul University Cerrahpasa Medical Faculty,
Department of Biochemistry, Istanbul, Turkey

Abstract

Normal body cells grow, divide, and die in an orderly fashion
through the life. Cancer appears when cells in a part of the body start to
grow out of control. Normal cells are transformed to cancer cells by a
process termed as carcinogenesis. The first step in the carcinogenesis is
DNA damage. In a normal cell, when DNA gets damaged the cell either
repairs the damage or directs itself to die by apoptosis (programmed cell
death). In a tumor cell, the damaged DNA is not repaired, and apoptosis
is inhibited. Therefore genetically damaged cell doesn't die like it should.
Instead, this cell keeps on dividing and makes new cells which contain
the same damaged DNA. Damaged DNA can be inherited, but genetic
heritage is responsible in approximately 5-10% of all cancers; 90-95% of
all cancers are derived from acquired genetic alterations. Environmental
effects which lead to mutations and/or epigenetic changes on target genes
are major risk factors for cancer. Lifestyle-related factors such as
nutritional habits, smoking, overexposure to sunlight, working conditions,
lack of exercise and stress are integral environmental factors.
Environmental factors are classified as physical, chemical and biological

---

[*] Email:yldz.dincer@gmail.com

carcinogens. This chapter provides an inside look to these factors and associated mechanisms involved in cancer development.

Introduction

Cancer is a major burden of disease worldwide. Its incidence increases not only in industrialized countries but also in developing countries day by day. Beyond individual suffering, the economic burden of cancer therapy to community is heavy. Every year millions of people are diagnosed as cancer and more than half of the cancer patients die from it despite the current improved methods of early detection, surgery and therapy. Cancer is the second major cause of death in the world after cardiovascular diseases. Although humans of all ages develop cancer, its incidence increases with age. Many of the people keep on living after developing the disease. Other than age, cancer incidence changes depending on sex, race, geographic settlement, workplace, socio-economic status, lifestyle, nutritional habits, smoking, alcohol consumption, hormonal and immunological factors and presence of precancerous pathologies.

Cancer can be defined as a relatively autonomous growth of tissue. A tumor is made up of billions of cells originating from an initial cell proliferating clonally. Cancer was mentioned for the first time by Hippocrates as 'karkinos'. In the 2nd century, Galeno used the word 'neoplasia'. He described it as the growth of body area adverse to nature. Breast tumefaction was cited in Edwin Smith's papyruses in 17th century. The causal relationship between environmental materials and tumor development was firstly noticed by English surgeon Percivall Pott in 1775. Genetic basis of neoplasia was determined for the first time in 1914 by Boveri who described the somatic mutation in cancer cells. Advances in molecular genetics have provided a better understanding of the carcinogenesis. In the last 50-60 years considerable improvement have been made in the perception of the cellular and molecular mechanisms underlying autonomolus growth of tissue. Especially, important improvements have been made between 1980 and 1990 by molecular studies on proto-oncogenes and tumor suppressor genes. It was disclosed that genetic heritage is responsible in nearly 5-10% of all cancer cases; 90-95% of the cancers are caused by environmental factors; and presence of environmental factors expedites the development of cancer in subjects with genetic heritage [1-3].

Cell proliferation takes place as result of cell division cycles which include synthesis phase (S), mitosis phase (M) and gaps (G0, G1, G2) (Figure 1). The proliferation of normal cells is regulated by growth promoting proto-oncogenes and compensated by growth inhibiting tumor suppressor genes. Phases of the cell division cycles are regulated by growth factors, cytokines, cyclines and cyclin-dependent kinases. Proto-oncogenes are the genes encoding growth factors, and all proteins involved in their signal transduction. Cancer appears when proto-oncogenes are activated and tumor suppressor genes are inactivated. Proto-oncogenes are activated to oncogenes by various mechanisms such as promoter or enhancer insertion, chromosomal translocations, gene amplification and mutations. These genetic alterations may be inherited or acquired. Now that cancer is derived from alterations in the genes which are involved in the regulation of cellular proliferation and differentiation, carcinogenesis should be evaluated in two dimensions: 1). Molecular mechanisms in carcinogenesis and 2). Environmental factors in carcinogenesis.

Molecular Mechanisms in Carcinogenesis

Cell dividing starts with embryonic development and goes on during the life. Tissues and organs are formed by differentiation of fastly growing embryonic cells. Cell proliferation is crucial for the maintenance of integrity of tissues and organs and is under tight control. When growth factors encoded by proto-oncogenes bind to their cellular receptors, a signal occurs and signal transduction mechanism is triggered to stimulate DNA synthesis. In requirement of limitation of growth, products of tumor suppressor genes generate a signal to inhibit DNA synthesis by triggering various mechanisms. When DNA is damaged, tumor suppressor proteins arrest cell cycle, thus give time to cell for repair of the damaged DNA. If DNA escapes from repair or repair capacity is overwhelmed due to extensive DNA damage, apoptosis (programmed cell death) is triggered by tumor suppressor proteins, and thus mitosis of genetically damaged cell is blocked. The tumour suppressor proteins p53, p21 and Rb play pivotal roles in cellular protection against carcinogenesis by blocking cell cycle at the G1 phase. Best studied and the most prominent tumour suppressor gene is p53. When DNA is damaged p53 interrupts the cell cycle at G1 phase and goes for a repair. If damage is too extensive p53 induces apoptosis in order to maintain the stability of genome [4]. p53 can be described as the guardian of the genome.

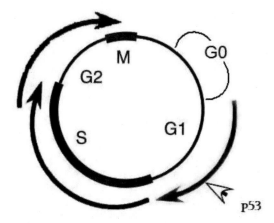

Figure 1.Cell cycle.

The loss of p53 during carcinogenesis can predispose preneoplastic cells to accumulate additional mutations by blocking the normal apoptotic response to DNA damage.

Carcinogenesis is a complex and multistage process. Many changes occur in the transcriptional activity of genes associated with many critical cellular processes during the malign transformation. Primary target genes in carcinogenesis are proto-oncogenes, tumor suppressor genes, DNA repair genes, apoptosis-related genes and the genes involved in regulation of cell cycle. Environmental carcinogens are capable of changing cell metabolism via genetic and epigenetic alterations.

Changes at the Genetic Level

Physical and chemical carcinogens are able to interact DNA to form base adducts. Some of these modified bases cause mispairing during the replication unless repaired, and subsequently lead to somatic mutations. Mutations in crucial genes may change the function of the gene products and lead to loss of the control on cellular growth. Results of the in vitro studies revealed that activation of one proto-oncogene or loss of one tumor suppressor gene was not enough to promote carcinogenesis; many alterations in various target genes should accumulate for cancer development. Indeed, cancer development requires many years. In human tumors, many activated oncogenes and two or more lost/inactivated tumor suppressor genes have been determined. The best evidence about this subject has been obtained in colorectal cancer studies. Each mutation associated with each step of the colorectal carcinogenesis has been clearly defined. Mutations can appear through deletions, frame shift or by base substitutions. Mutations cause various cellular changes translated into aberrant protein expression and changes in control of the cell cycle.

Changes at the Epigenetic Level

Recently, it was determined that genetic alteration is not the unique pathway for carcinogenesis, epigenetic factors are also responsible for cancer development. The term 'epigenetics' refers to altered transcriptional activity of a gene without any change in its primary base sequence. Epigenetic factors involve alterations in DNA methylation status and specific histone modifications such as acetylation, deacetylation and methylation.

DNA methylation is an important epigenetic determinant of gene expression. In general, increased methylation at CpG sites in the promoter region of certain genes causes gene transcriptional silencing. Silencing of the tumor suppressor genes, DNA repair genes and genes involved in apoptosis by promoter hypermethylation contribute to multistage process of carcinogenesis. Furthermore, genome-wide hypomethylation may increase mutation rates and thus may cause genome instability. Methylation of DNA is carried out by DNA methyltransferases.

These enzymes catalyze the transfer of a methyl group from S-adenosylmethionine to the 5'-carbon of cytosine within CpG dinucleotide. Various forms of DNA methyltransferases have been determined but DNA methyltransferase 1, DNA methyltransferase 3a and DNA methyltransferase 3b are critical in DNA methylation reactions. 5-methylcytosine is a heritable modification, and it also contributes to carcinogenesis by increasing mutation rate. 5'-methylcytosine promotes the deamination of cytosine to uracil. Spontaneous deamination of 5'-methylcytosine is 2-4 fold higher than those of cytosine [5].

Increased expression of DNA methyltransferase 1 has been determined in early and late stages of cancer. Many genes in tumor cells have been demonstrated to contain alterations in their DNA methylation status. p16, RASSF1 and O^6MGMT genes (p16 and RASSF1 are tumor suppressor genes, O^6MGMT is a DNA repair gene) have been suggested as common targets of promoter hypermethylation in lung cancer. In a prospective study, hypermethylation in promoter region of p16 and O^6MGMT genes in sputum has been found to be strongly associated with lung cancer risk. The aberrant methylation in promoter of O^6MGMT gene in oral rinse from patients with oral squamous cell carcinoma have been determined. In head and neck cancer, promoter hypermethylation and decreased expression in p16, O^6MGMT and RASSF1 genes have been reported. Promoter hypermethylation in RASSF1 gene and in O^6MGMT gene have been found to be associated with ovarian cancer and glioblastoma, respectively. It has been determined that klotho, a novel tumor suppressor gene, was silenced through promoter hypermethylation in gastric cancer.

In another recent investigation, promoter methylation in RASSF1 and SFRP1 (a tumor suppressor gene) genes have been examined in exfoliated epithelial cells in the breast milk obtained from each breast of women with a history of a non-proliferative benign breast biopsy versus reference group consisted of women for whom a breast biopsy was not required. Mean methylation scores for RASSF1 has been found to be significantly higher in the biopsy group than in the reference group. A comparison between the biopsied and non-biopsied breasts of the biopsy group revealed higher mean methylation in the biopsied breast for both SFRP1 and RASSF1. These results show that women had a non-proliferative benign breast mass in the past may be at increased risk of developing breast cancer based on having hypermethylated promoter for tumor suppressor genes. Taken together, recent studies disclosed the importance of promoter hypermethylation in certain target genes in cancer etiology and addressed the epigenetic factors as promising biomarker for assessing cancer risk [6-14].

Another key mechanism in epigenetic pathways is histone modifications. The mammalian genome is comprised of DNA, which is tightly packaged into a nucleoprotein structure named as chromatin. The basic subunit of chromatin is the nucleosome. Nucleosome consists of approximately 147 base pairs of DNA wrapped around an octameric histone core which includes a dimer of heterotetrameric histones H2A, H2B, H3, and H4. A linker histone, H1, is present in the region of inter nucleosome linker DNA and have an effect on nucleosome interactions and chromatin structure. Histones are dynamic molecules that provide physical support to DNA and are involved in the regulation of replication, transcription and repair. Histones possess flexible tails which are target to post-translational biochemical modifications such as acetylation, methylation, and phosphorylation.

These modifications occur on specific amino acids by the reactions catalyzed by numerous different histone modifying enzymes in response to various external and internal stimulatory signals. Covalent modifications of N- or C-terminal histone tails alter chromatin structure and serve to recruit or to exclude protein complexes from DNA. Acetylation and methylation are the most recognized modifications. Acetylation/deacetylation of histone tails is a common mechanism involved in regulation of gene expression. Acetylation decreases the affinity of histones to DNA and leads an open chromatin conformation to allow gene transcription, and histone deacetylation causes to closed chromatin. In other words, histone acetylation maintains chromatin in a transcriptionally active state, whereas histone deacetylation leads transcriptional silencing. Specific enzymes selectively remove the histone tail modifications. Histone acetyltransferases and histone deacetyltransferases balance the acetylation of histone tails. DNA methyltransferases direct the binding of histone deacetylases and some specific proteins such as methyl-CpG binding proteins to hypermethylated regions of the chromatin. These proteins form a complex that prevents access of the transcriptional machinery to the promoter region. It is thought that histone methylation may also be associated either with transcriptional activation or repression. Histone modifications are implicated in genomic imprinting, X chromosome inactivation, embryonic stem cell development, and differentiation in normal cells. Disruption of these processes may lead to carcinogenesis. In malignant cells, genome-wide histone modifications were found to be altered in accordance with alterations in DNA methylation status. Alterations in the expression of histone acetyltransferases, histone deacetyltransferases, histone methyltransferases and histone demethylaseshave been associated with carcinogenesis. Aberrated histone modifications frequently occur in tumor cells and they end with changes in their levels and distribution at gene promoters, gene coding regions and repetitive DNA sequences. Interestingly, it has been determined that the same repressive histone marks were defined in certain genes with tumor-suppression effect which was not silenced by DNA methylation. Locus specific alterations in histone modifications may have adverse effects on expression of nearby genes. Alterations in global levels of specific histone modifications determined in cancer cells generate an additional layer of epigenetic heterogeneity at the cellular level in tumor tissues. It was suggested that in general, increased prevalence of cells with lower global levels of histone modifications is prognostic of poorer clinical outcome such as increased risk of tumor recurrence and/or decreased survival possibility. Prognostic utility of histone modifications have been demonstrated independently for multiple cancers including those of breast, ovary, prostate, lung, kidney, and pancreas [15-19].

Environmental Factors in Carcinogenesis

Only a small fraction of cancers is attributed to germline mutations in cancer-related genes. Germline mutations in more than 20 different genes were reported as hereditary traits increasing susceptibility to cancer. The tumor suppressor genes p53 and adenomatous polyposis coli (APC); DNA repair genes BRCA1 and BRCA2 are the genes recognized to be responsible for hereditary cancers. Germline mutations are frequently determined in subjects with a family history or those with second malignancies. Majority of the cancers are derived from acquired genetic alterations formed by environmental factors. Frequency of exposure to environmental carcinogens in daily life is determined by job, workplace, dietary habits and lifestyle. Environmental factors play an important role in the etiology of cancer by modulating important changes in target genes. Alterations in cellular genome after a carcinogenic exposure may result in malignancy if apoptosis is prevented and the immune system fails to eliminate the transformed cells. Environmental influences leading mutations and/or epigenetic changes on target genes are considered major risk factors for cancer. Their roles in tumor formation have been widely supported by epidemiological and experimental animal studies. The environmental factors responsible for cancer development are classified as physical, chemical, biological carcinogens. Lifestyle-related factors such as nutritional habits (food preservation and preparation, ingestion of certain foods, food contamination by mycotoxins), smoking, alcohol consumption, excess exposure to sunlight, workplace, lack of exercise, stress are themselves integral environmental factors. Unhealthy lifestyle habits are responsible for higher incidence of certain types of cancer. Although the role of lifestyle-related factors in cancer development is known, they are generally ignored. Differences in the incidence and tumor type among different ethnic and geographical populations emphasize the influence of environmental factors in carcinogenesis. These differences are derived from different lifestyle factors and habits in different cultures living in different areas of the world. Best defined examples are differences in frequency of certain types of cancer between Japanese and Western populations. The rates of breast and prostate cancer are a few times higher in Western populations as compared to Japanese.

The rate of gastric cancer in Japan is six times higher than those in Western countries. However, the incidence of gastric cancer decreased considerably in Japanese people who migrated to Western countries. An important increase in the incidence of breast cancer determined in the Japanese women only one generation upon migrating to USA [20, 21]. It seems that changes in environment may be related with major shifts in cancer prevalence.

Several lines of evidence indicate the role of diet and nutrition in carcinogenesis. Carcinogenicity of N-nitrosamines available in beer, cheese, smoked fish and processed meat products; heterocyclic amines produced during the cooking of meat; alcohol and tobacco were recognized long time ago. In some parts of Asia a very high incidence of gastrointestinal system cancers is observed. This is thought to be derived from frequent consumption of smoked fish and smoked vegetables which are sources of high levels of N-nitrosamines. Colon cancer incidence is also high in Western countries depending on the consumption of red meat. Especially processed meat products such as sausages, bacon and ham are the major sources of N-nitroso compounds. Epidemiological studies show that countries where people eat more red meat are also the countries where colon cancer incidence is high [22]. On the other hand, colon cancer incidence is very low in people living in tropical regions of Africa. This is attributed to high fiber containing diet that is common in these regions, because fibers lead quickly to excretion of potential carcinogens from colon. Soy products frequently consumed in Asia contain high levels of phytoestrogens which are non-steroidal plant-derived compounds with a similar structure to endogenous estrogens. Although discussed so much because of inconsistent data, frequent consumption of soy foods is suggested due to low incidence of breast and ovary cancers observed in women living in Asia [22-24].

Obesity is a well-defined risk factor for certain types of cancer and there is a correlation between obesity and cancer risk. It is known that excessive calories and high fat intake increases the risk of certain cancers such as prostate, colon and breast. A high fat intake stimulates the synthesis and secretion of bile acids by the liver into the intestine. High concentrations of bile acids in colon stimulates bacterial activity to produce carcinogenic metabolites. Accumulation of excess fat in adipose tissue induces the conversion of androstenedione to estrogen which increases breast cancer risk. In the case of normal fat intake, the kind and amount of dietary fatty acids have been found to be related with cancer development. Animal fat rich in saturated fatty acids and plant-derived n-6 polyunsaturated fatty acids derived from corn and sun-flower are suggested to increase cancer risk; n-3 polyunsaturated fatty acids found in fish oil and n-9 monounsaturated fatty acids found in olive oil are suggested to protect against cancer [25].

Physical Agents in Carcinogenesis

The major physical agents causing cancer development are ionizing radiation and UV.

Ionizing Radiation

Whenever the energy of a photon exceeds the energy required to remove an electron from a molecule, the molecule is converted to an ion as a result of the collision. γ–rays, X-rays and high- energy electrons (β-particles), high-energy neutrons and α–particles are sufficiently energetic to ionize biomolecules and these are called ionizing radiation. Carcinogenic effect of ionizing radiation has been evidenced after long-term investigations and observations on survivors of atom bomb in Japan, people exposed to nuclear accidents and people frequently exposed to X-rays for diagnosis and follow up. It has also been evidenced in cancer patients that after a successive radiotherapy secondary malignancy may appear within five years due to ionizing radiation-mediated damage of the healthy cells.

The impact of ionizing radiation to cells may be directly or by oxidative stress, indirectly. Direct effect appears in the form of DNA strand breaks derived from collision of radiation energy and DNA. This type of DNA damage is lethal rather than become mutagenic. Indirect effect is formed by interaction of DNA and cellular molecules excited by radiation energy. Majority of the damage done to cells by ionizing radiation is derived from oxidative stress via formation of hydroxyl radicals (OH·) which is the most effective reactive oxygen species. OH·readily attacks to all cellular molecules including DNA. OH·are generated when the water within the cell exposed to ionizing radiation, and then secondary reactions lead to increased formation of other reactive oxygen species. As a result of OH·attack to DNA strand breaks and base modifications occur. Extensive strand breaks leads to activation of apoptosis, and thus cell with heavily damaged DNA undergoes to death. Carcinogenic effect of ionizing radiation appears as a result of formation of mutagenic base modifications. Up to date a number of oxidatively modified bases have been identified. Some of these modified bases do not pair off during the DNA replication and cause frame shift mutations. Certain oxidized bases mismatch and lead to point mutations unless repaired before the replication. Among these modified bases, 8-hydroxydeoxyguanosine (8-OHdG) is the predominant lesion. It is formed through oxidation of guanine at the C8 position. 8-OHdG has a pro-mutagenic potential by mispairing with A residues, leading to an increased frequency of spontaneous G:C→T:A transversion. This mutation is generally observed in mutated proto-oncogenes and tumor suppressor genes. 8-OHdG residues on DNA are excised by repair enzymes, appear in the blood and are subsequently excreted in the urine. 8-OHdG levels in blood and urine are measured as a marker of oxidative DNA damage. A variety of environmental agents including ionizing radiation were reported to increase 8-OHdG level in cellular DNA as well in blood and urine [26].

Recently, considerable interest has focused on oxidative modifications of RNA by reactive oxygen species. It has been evidenced that purified RNA was much more susceptible to oxidation than DNA. Oxidative damage to RNA causes base and ribose modifications, base excision and strand breaks. Certain oxidative RNA modifications including 8-OHdG, 8-hydroxyadenine and 5-hydroxycytosine have been determined. Oxidative damage to RNA may potentially leads to mistakes in protein synthesis and may also exert non-acute lethal impact. Oxidative RNA damage has been shown in several neurodegenerative diseases and it is still under investigation for carcinogenesis [26-28].

UV

UV is a well-documented risk factor for skin cancer. UV light with a 290-320 nm wavelength is insufficiently energetic to ionize biomolecules. They exert their carcinogenic effects by forming dimers between adjacent thymines, and by creating a basic, apurinic/apyrimidinic sites. Beyond these genetic changes, some epigenetic changes have also been identified as cellular response to UV radiation. Post-translational modifications triggered by UV irradiation in membrane, cytoplasma and nuclear compartments have been evidenced. UV irradiation causes dimerization of insulin like growth factor receptor and epidermal growth factor receptor in cellular plasma membrane. UV irradiation was implicated in the induction of signaling cascades including protein kinase C, mitogen activated protein kinase and Janus kinase within the cytosol. These cascades are thought to be induced by UV-mediated alterations in downstream effectors such as jun, fos, p53 and nuclear factor κB. One of the better-characterized kinases activated by UV irradiation is Janus kinase. Janus kinase has been found to be persistently activated in apoptosis induced by UV. Activated Janus kinase phosphorylates key regulatory transcription factors such as c-jun, ATF2 and p53. Phosphorylation of c-Jun by activated Janus kinase protects it from ubiquitination, thus prolongs its half-life and impact [29-32].

Biological Agents in Carcinogenesis

Accumulating data have shown the association with bacterial/viral infections and certain types of cancer.

Bacterial Infections

Epidemiological evidences indicate that schistosoma haemotobium infection is associated with squamous cell carcinoma of the urinary bladder. Similarly, an association between helicobacter pylori and increased risk for gastric cancer is determined. Bacteria are not capable of damaging DNA directly. Cancer arises as a result of immune response to these infectious agents, especially in case of chronic infections. An enormous amount of reactive oxygen/nitrogen species are produced during the respiratory burst in phagocytic cells. These reactive molecules cause oxidative stress. Oxidative stress is a state characterized by an imbalance between the production of reactive oxygen species and the detoxification of these reactive intermediates. Oxidative stress plays a fundamental role in the initiation, promotion and progression of tumor by causing DNA strand breakages, base modifications, and chromosome abnormalities [33, 34].

Viral Infections

In addition to induce immune response, many viruses contain oncogenes which are responsible for malign transformation in host cells. Viruses classified as RNA tumor viruses have single stranded RNA genome and RNA-directed DNA polymerase activity, reverse transcriptase. On infection, single stranded RNA viral genome and reverse transcriptase enter the host cell, and reverse transcriptase catalyzes the synthesis of a DNA strand complementary to the viral RNA. The same enzyme degrades the formed RNA-DNA hybrid and incorporates the viral DNA into DNA of the host cell. Therefore, viral DNA is integrated to host cell genome, and viral oncogene is expressed by host cell. The first discovered retrovirus contributing tumor formation is Raus sarcoma virus which contains *src*oncogene and causes sarcomas in chickens. Proto-oncogenes found in normal mammalian cells are similar in base sequence to the viral oncogenes. Viruses not having oncogenes may also cause cancer. Incorporated viral DNA may activate a nearby proto-oncogene in the host cell genome, and may induce carcinogenesis although virus does not contain oncogenes. One of the most studied and well-characterized carcinogenic viruses is human papilloma virus (HPV). HPV incorporates its viral DNA into the host genome. Viral oncoproteins encoded by the E6 and E7 genes are responsible for HPV-mediated carcinogenesis. E6 and E7 proteins form complexes with p53 and Rb proteins which are involved in checkpoint of cell cycle. Formed complexes prevent activation of p53 and Rb [35, 36]. Infection with human papilloma virus has been determined to be associated with most types of uterine and cervical cancer. However, HPV infection by itself is not enough for development of cervical cancer; combination of HPV infection and accumulated genetic alterations leads to malignant progression.

Epidemiological and clinical studies show a strong association between Epstein Barr virus and Burkitt lymphoma; hepatitis B virus (HBV), hepatitis C virus (HCV) and hepatocellular carcinoma; human T-cell leukemia virus and T-cell leukemia ; human herpes virus 8 and Kaposi's sarcoma. HBV and HCV are hepatotropic viruses and are responsible for 80-90% of hepatocellular cancer cases worldwide. When HBV-DNA integrated to host cell DNA, site of viral integration may be nearby to the target genes involved in cellular signaling pathways. HBV-DNA integration to host cell genome has been shown to lead chromosomal deletions, as found at the chromosomal region 17p11.2-12 causing the loss of the p53 gene; and chromosomal disruptions or translocations resulting in genetic instability. HCV lacks capacity of integrating itself into the host cell genome and does not carry oncogenes. It exerts its carcinogenic effect by an indirect mechanism based on chronic liver damage, inflammation and cellular regeneration [37-39].

All of these events may cause cell transformation, but it should be kept in mind that cancer does not arise until a dysfunctional immune surveillance system is unable to prevent tumor development. This situation is generally observed in subjects with chronic states of immunosuppression such as patients receiving therapy to prevent allograft rejection, those with HIV and individuals with congenital immune disorders. Generally all these subjects have a higher risk of cancer development.

Chemical Agents in Carcinogenesis

The relationship between chemical substances and tumor development was recognized for the first time in 1775 by occurrence of cancerous changes in the skin of the scrotum of London chimney sweeps as a result of repeated contamination by soot. In the same century, the association between the increased rate of nasal mucosa cancer and long-term exposure of snuff was determined. In 1890, a high incidence of urinary bladder cancer in rubber and chemical industry workers was stated in Europe. By the end of the 19th century, it was obvious that occupational exposure to certain chemicals causes cancer [1, 40-42]. After that, experimental models were established to investigate carcinogenic effects of occupational substances. The first experimental work on chemical-induced carcinogenesis was performed by Yamagiwa et al. [43] in 1915. A chemical substance is considered carcinogenic when its administration to laboratory animals induces a significant increase in the incidence of tumor development as compared to animals which are not exposed to the substance. Yamagiwa et al. rubbed rabbit ears with coal tar to induce carcinoma. Meantime, carcinogenesis in lung, liver, kidney, pancreas and urinary bladder were examined by various investigators. In 1947, carcinogenic potencies of polycyclic aromatic hydrocarbons and croton oil in skin carcinogenesis in mice were investigated by Beremblum and Shubik [44]. It was determined that when applied in low doses, separately, none of the substances have carcinogenic potency but when they mixed, they induced neoplastic development. The order of exposure of the substances was the main determinant for carcinogenesis; neoplasias developed only in the case of polycyclic aromatic hydrocarbons were used first and then croton oil. Authors suggested two phases in carcinogenesis as initiation and promotion, and one or two genetic changes in these phases. In 1954, the term progression was introduced by Foulds [45] who studied on chemically induced breast carcinogenesis in female mice. In early experimental studies, tumor development was believed to be derived from interaction of carcinogenic substances with proteins in specific tissues. After the discovery of DNA structure by Watson and Crick, increasing evidence indicated the association between DNA binding capacity of chemical substances and their carcinogenic potency. In vitro studies, animal models and epidemiological researches revealed that cancer induction by chemical substances involves three steps defined as initiation, promotion and progression.

Initiation - This is the fast, irreversible step where DNA damage is formed by chemicals as well physical agents. DNA damage can be repaired but if cellular division happens before the DNA repair process, the damage becomes permanent. DNA with unrepaired damage undergoes replication, mutation occurs, and then a mutated, initiated cell is produced. The initiated cell is not a neoplastic cell, mutations induce proliferation but do not effect differentiation. The initiated cell is similar to remaining cells. Increased proliferation does not confer time for repair of damaged DNA, thus initiated cells have less time for the repairing process. In addition, during cell proliferation mutations may be acquired due to misrepair of damaged DNA. The initiated cells can remain latent for weeks, months or years, alternatively they can grow autonomously and clonally. Development of neoplasia depends on dose of carcinogenic agent. High dose enhances the incidence and multiplicity of neoplasias and decreases the latent period of its manifestation. Cell proliferation is essential for this stage. The clonal expansion of initiated cells is a consequence of a mitogenic process caused by increased numbers of new cells and inhibition of apoptosis which exterminates initiated cells [1].

Beyond an external carcinogenic agent, initiation may be started by spontaneous DNA damage which occurs during normal DNA metabolism. Deamination of bases, depurination/depyrimidination, formation of a basic sites, errors in DNA replication occur every day in all cells. However, these damages are generally repaired before the replication and this type of initiation is less common when compared to induced initiation [1]. The production of the initiated cell can occur through interaction with physical carcinogens such as UV light and radiation in addition to chemical carcinogens.

Promotion - Following the formation of the initiated cell, chemical substances can cause the selective clonal growth of this initiated cell through the process of tumor promotion. This step involves the expansion of the initiated cell to a focal lesion. The tumor promotion is not a direct DNA damaging process, but involves modulation of gene expression that results with increased mutations, increased cell number through cell division and/or decreased apoptotic cell death [46]. Following continual cell proliferation, additional mutations may be acquired in preneoplastic cells. This results in the formation of neoplasms. Epigenetic mechanisms are also involved in promotion step. Most important effect of promoter substances is mitogenesis. Some promoter substances are specific for a specific tissue, but others act simultaneously on several tissues. In order to exert their effect promoter substances must be available for weeks, months and years in the target tissue. Promotion is a reversible step. After disappearance of a promoter substance, cell proliferation can decrease. This regression is generally attributed to apoptosis. Experimental studies show that prolonged exposure and high doses of all promoter substances (e.g. asbestos, arsenic, benzene and phenobarbital) induce neoplasias without initiation (1, 47, 48). Lesions histopathologically identified between initiation and promotion are termed as preneoplastic lesions or benign neoplasias [1, 47, 48].

Progression - In this last step of carcinogenesis, preneoplastic lesions are transformed into malign lesions. Progression step involves genetic and epigenetic mechanisms. Progression is characterised by irreversibility, additional DNA damage, genetic instability, faster growth, acquisition of the ability of invasion and metastization. Angiogenesis which appears as a result of epigenetic alterations is associated with progression. Morphological and biochemical alterations occur. Purine and pyrimidine biosynthesis, DNA replication, protein synthesis and glucose utilization increase in neoplastic cells. During progression, cell proliferation is independent from the presence of stimulus [47, 49].

Initiator and promoter substances are generally non-polar lipophilic molecules. Minority of them can react with DNA directly. Majority of chemical carcinogens, termed as pro-carcinogen, gain the ability to interact with DNA after metabolic activation. Metabolic activation reactions occurs predominantly in the liver by microsomal cytochrome P450 system.

Metabolic Activation of Chemical Carcinogens

Detoxification of various xenobiotics such as drugs, chemicals and metabolization of non-polar endogenous metabolites are achieved by phase I and phase II reactions predominantly in liver. Phase I reactions involve oxidation (generally hydroxylation), reduction, epoxidation, deamination, desulphuration and dehallogenation. In phase II reactions, hydroxylated chemicals by the phase I reactions are converted to more polar molecules by conjugation with glucuronate, sulfate, amino acids or acetate in order to be excreted by either renal or biliary-intestinal system. Glutathione S-transferases, N-acetyltransferases, UDP-glucuronosyltransferases, sulfotransferases are the major enzymes involved in phase II reactions.

Cytochrome P450 system is a family of closely similar proteins. They take part in various metabolic reactions other than detoxification process. Several hundred members of cytochrome P450 are identified. Each cytochrome P450 enzyme has a different substrate specificity. Cytochrome P450 enzymes catalyze hydroxylation reactions in which one of the two oxygen atoms of O_2 is incorporated into the chemical molecule and the other being reduced to water. Unfortunately, hydroxylation of some chemical molecules by this way converts them to electrophilic metabolites that are readily interacting with DNA to form covalent chemical-DNA adducts. DNA abundantly contains nucleophilic sites and thus, a well target for electrophilic attacks. The formation of DNA adducts constitutes the first step of carcinogenesis unless repaired before the replication. Cytochrome P450-mediated chemical carcinogenesis, especially role of cytochrome P448 in polycyclic aromatic hydrocarbon-mediated carcinogenesis is well defined. It is determined that depending on its chemical structure, the same enzyme may activate one chemical whereas deactivate another [50]. However, all of these knowledge were obtained from either in vitro or experimental animal studies. Although the process of carcinogenesis is similar for humans and experimental animals, there are qualitative and quantitative differences between them. These differences may cause to incorrect interpretations when animal models are used in investigation. It should be marked that different chemical substances may change the speed of the process, frequency of mutation and rate of cellular growth in man.

One of the causes of interindividual differences in cancer development is genetic polymorphisms in phase I and phase II enzymes. People with a high activity of phase I and a low activity of phase II enzymes have a higher possibility of producing electrophilic intermediate metabolites, exhibiting more DNA damage and finally of cancer development [51]. In addition, phase I and phase II enzymes are inducible and their activity may change depending on age, gender, race, diet, alcohol consumption and presence of liver and kidney diseases.

Classification of Chemical Carcinogens Depending on Their Action Mechanisms

Chemical carcinogens are classified as genotoxic and non-genotoxic [1]. Genotoxic chemical carcinogens exert their effects by forming covalent DNA adducts as mentioned above. Polycyclic aromatic hydrocarbons, aromatic amines and amides, N-nitroso compounds, aminoazo dyes, anticancer drugs, and aflatoxin B1 constitute this group. Non-genotoxic chemical carcinogens act as promoter. They are tissue-and species-specific. They do not need metabolic activation and do not directly interact with DNA [52]. They potentiate the effects of genotoxic chemical carcinogens, modulate cellular growth and death. Non-genotoxic chemical carcinogens are classified as cytotoxic and mitogenic.

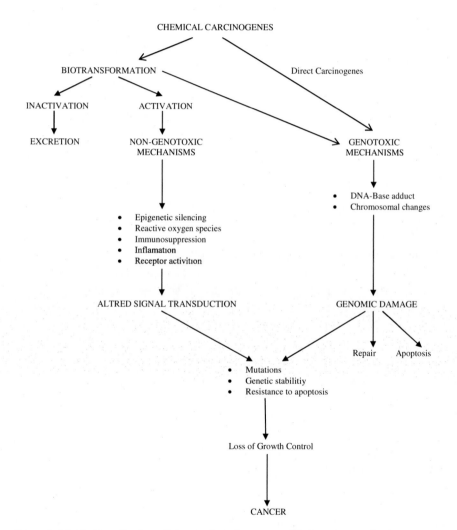

Figure 2. Metabolic activation of chemical carcinogens and their action mechanisms [Adapted from reference 1].

Table 1. Chemical carcinogens and affected organs

Group	Chemical compound	Affected organs
Polycyclic aromatic hydrocarbons	Benzo[α] pyrene Polychlorinated biphenyls	Stomach, colon, lung, liver, skin
Aromatic amines/ amides	2-Acetylaminofluorene, aniline, 4-Aminobiphenyl, 2-Naphthylamine	Stomach, colon, breast, prostate Liver, urinary bladder
N-nitroso compounds	N-nitrosodimethylamine Methylnitrosourea	Liver, lung, stomach, colon larynx, esophagus, kidney, urinary bladder
Aminoazo dyes	O-Aminoazotoluene	Liver, lung, urinary bladder
Inorganic compounds	Asbestos, arsenic, cadmium nickel, chrome	Skin, liver, lung, kidney prostate
Anticancer drugs	Alkylating agents, dactinomycin	Leukemia
Others	Alcohol, aflatoxin B1 phorbol esters	Oropharynx, larynx, esophagus liver, breast, colon

Cytotoxic carcinogens cause cell death in susceptible tissues when used as high doses. After death of some cells, nearby cells exhibit a compensatory increase in cell division through regenerative procedures and hyperplasia occurs.

In addition, remnants of the necrosed cells are phagocyte by immune system cells.

During this process, oxidative damage occurs due to increased formation of reactive oxygen and nitrogen species. Oxidative DNA lesions cause either mutations or cell death if they are not repaired. Metals such as arsenic and cadmium are well defined cytotoxic carcinogens.

Mitogenic carcinogens induce cell proliferation via interaction with specific cellular receptors. Phorbol esters and dioxins are in this group. In order to promote their activity, mitogenic compounds must be present at certain concentrations in target tissue (Figure 2) [1].

Chemical carcinogens can have additional synergic effects if simultaneous exposure occurs. One of the best characterized examples is the synergy between smoking and chronic alcohol consumption. Alcohol induces cytochrome P450 system. Induction of cytochrome P450 results increases metabolic activation of tobacco-specific carcinogens as well as increasing production of reactive oxygen species. By inducing cytochrome P450, alcohol increases the incidence of the lung cancer development in smokers compared to non-alcoholic smokers. Likely, the synergy between smoking and asbestos exposure accelerates development of lung cancer as a result of chronic inflammation-mediated oxidative DNA damage and compensatory cell proliferation.

Chemical carcinogens such as polycyclic aromatic hydrocarbons, aromatic amines/ amides, aminoazo dyes are used in textile, dye, cosmetic, food, rubber and chemical industries. N-nitroso compounds and their precursors are found in processed, smoked meat and fish products, beer, cigarette, even in drinking water and some rubber products. Aflatoxin B1 is a mycotoxine produced by Aspergillusflavus or Aspergillusparasiticus that can infect peanuts, but also infects tree nuts and grains stored in humid mediums. Groups of the chemical carcinogens and affected organs are shown in the Table 1 [1].

Conclusion

Objective of this chapter was to review the current knowledge available on carcinogenesis and to provide a basis for the following chapters. Cancer is a disease characterized by loss of control on cellular growth, invasiveness and metastasis. Minority of the cancers are related with heredity, and cancer can be caused by mainly environmental factors in relation with life-style. The first step in the carcinogenesis is always DNA damage. Physical, chemical and biologic agents encountered during the human life, depending of life -style, damage or alter DNA. Although carcinogenic impacts of some environmental risk factors are well known, avoiding from these factors is generally ignored. Understanding the carcinogenic mechanisms may be convincing for exclusion of these factors from our daily lives. Thus, consciously elimination of some risk factors may reduce a portion of diet-related, occupational and environmental life-style cancers.

Acknowledgments

The author thanks Onur Baykara for English revision, and Armagan Caglayan for her assistance in the organisation of references, figures and tables.

References

[1]   Oliveira, PA; Colaço, A; Chaves, R; Guedes-Pinto, H; De-La-Cruz, PLF; Lopes, C. Chemical Carcinogenesis. *An Acad. Bras. Cienc.,* 2007 79(4), 593-616.

[2]   Weisburger, JH. Carcinogenicity and mutagenicity testing, then and now. *Mutat. Res.,* 1999 437, 105-112.

[3]   Anand, P; Kunnumakara, AB; Sundaram, C; Harikumar, KB; Tharakan, ST. Cancer is a preventable disease that requires major lifestyle changes. *Pharm. Res.,* 2008 25(9), 2007-2116.

[4]   Hanawalt, PC; Ford, JM; Lloyd, DR. Functional characterization of global genomic DNA repair and its implications for cancer. *Mutat. Res.,* 2003 544, 107-114.

[5]   Pfeifer, GP; Tang, M; Denissenko, MF. Mutation hotspots and DNA methylation. *Curr. Top Microbiol. Immunol.,* 2000 249, 1-19.

[6]   Alber, GAJ; Brock, MV; Samet, JM. Epidemiology of lung cancer: looking to the future. *J. Clin. Oncol. ,*2005 23(14), 3175-3185.

[7]   Belinsky, SA; Klinge, DM; Dekker, JD; Smith, MW; Bocklage, TJ; Gilliland, FD; Crowell, RE; Karp, DD; Stidley, CA; Picchi, MA. Gene promoter methylation in plasma and sputum increases with lung cancer risk. *Clin. Cancer Res.,*2005 11(18), 6505-6511.

[8]   Nagata, S; Hamada, T; Yamada, N; Yokoyama, S; Kitamoto, S; Kanmura, Y; Nomura, M; Kamikawa, Y; Yonezawa, S, Sugihara, K. Aberrant DNA methylation of tumor-related genes in oral rinse: A noninvasive method for detection of oral squamous cell carcinoma. *Cancer,* 2012 doi: 10.1002/cncr.27417.

[9]   Demokan, S; Chuang, A; Suoğlu, Y; Ulusan, M; Yalnız, Z; Califano, JA; Dalay, N. Promoter methylation and loss of p16(INK4a) gene expression in head and neck cancer. Head Neck, 2011 doi: 10.1002/hed.21949.

[10] Koutsimpelas, D; Pongsapich, W; Heinrich, U; Mann, S; Mann, WJ; Brieger, J. Promoter methylation of MGMT, MLH1 and RASSF1A tumor suppressor genes in head and neck squamous cell carcinoma: pharmacological genome demethylation reduces proliferation of head and neck squamous carcinoma cells. Oncol. Rep., 2012 27(4), 1135-1141

[11] Cul'bová, M; Lasabová, Z; Stanclová, A; Tilandyová, P; Zúbor, P; Fiolka, R; Danko, J; Visnovský, J. Methylation of selected tumor-supressor genes in benign and malignant ovarian tumors. CeskaGynekol., 2011 76(4), 274-279.

[12] Cecener, G; Tunca, B; Egeli, U; Bekar, A; Tezcan, G; Erturk, E; Bayram, N; Tolunay, S. The promoter hypermethylation status of GATA6, MGMT and FHIT in glioblastoma. Cell Mol. Neurobiol., 2011.

[13] Wang, L; Wang, X; Wang, X; Jie, P; Lu, H; Zhang, S; Lin, X; Lam, EK; Cui, Y; Yu, J; Jin, H. Klotho is silenced through promoter hypermethylation in gastric cancer. Am. J. Cancer Res., 2011 1(1), 111-119.

[14] Browne, EP; Punska, EC; Lenington, S; Otis, CN; Anderton, DL; Arcaro, KF. Increased promoter methylation in exfoliated breast epithelial cells in women with a previous breast biopsy. Epigenetics, 2011 6(12), 1425-1435.

[15] Franco, R; Schoneveld, O; Georgakilas, AG; Panayiotidis, MI. Oxidative stress, DNA methylation and carcinogenesis. Cancer Lett., 2008 266(1), 6-11.

[16] Sharma, S; Kelly, TK; Jones, PA. Epigenetics in cancer. Carcinogenesis, 2010 31, 27–36.

[17] Jerónimo, C; Bastian, PJ; Bjartell, A; Carbone, GM; Catto, JW; Clark, SJ; Henrique, R; Nelson, WG; Shariat, SF. Epigenetics in prostate cancer: biologic and clinical relevance. Eur. Urol., 2011 60(4), 753-766.

[18] Fraga, MF; Ballestar, E; Villar-Garea, A. Loss of acetylation at Lys16 and trimethylation at Lys20 of histone H4 is a common hallmark of human cancer. Nat. Genet., 2005 37, 391–400.

[19] Kurdistani, SK. Histone modifications in cancer biology and prognosis. Prog. Drug. Res., 2011 67, 91-106.

[20] Iarc, L. Cancer incidence in five continents. IARC Scientific Publications, 1997 6.

[21] Kakizoe, T. Cancer statistics in Japan. FPCR publication, 1997 10.

[22] Santarelli, RL; Pierre, F; Corpet, DE. Processed meat and colorectal cancer: a review of epidemiologic and experimental evidence. *Nutr. Cancer,* 2008 60(2), 131-144.

[23] Shu, XO; Zheng, Y; Cai, H; Gu, K; Chen, Z; Zheng, W. Soy food intake and breast cancer survival. *JAMA,* 2009 302, 2437–2443.

[24] Bandera, EV; King, M; Chandran, U; Paddock, LE; Rodriguez-Rodriguez, L; Olson, SH. Phytoestrogen consumption from foods and supplements and epithelial ovarian cancer risk: a population-based case control study. *BMC Womens Health,* 2011 11, 40.

[25] López-Miranda, J; Pérez-Jiménez, F; Ros, E; De Caterina, R`; Badimón, L; Covas, MI; Escrich, E; Ordovás, JM; Soriguer, F; Abiá, R; de la Lastra, CA; Battino, M; Corella, D; Chamorro-Quirós, J; et al. Olive oil and health: summary of the II international conference on olive oil and health consensus report, Jaén and Córdoba (Spain). *Nutr. Metab. Cardiovasc. Dis.,* 2008 20(4), 284-294.

[26] Klaunig, JE; Wang, Z; Pu, X; Zhou, S. Oxidative stress and oxidative damage in chemical carcinogenesis. *Toxicol. Appl. Pharmacol.,* 2011 254(2), 86-99.

[27] Li, Z; Wu, J; Deleo, CJ.RNA damage and surveillance under oxidative stress. *IUBMB Life,* 58(10), 581-588.

[28] Nunomura, A; Moreira, PI; Takeda, A; Smith, MA; Perry, G. Oxidative RNA damage and neurodegeneration. *Curr. Med. Chem.,*2007 14(28), 2968-2975.

[29] Minamoto, T; Mai, M; Ronai, Z. Environmental factors as regulators and effectors of multistep carcinogenesis. *Carcinogenesis,* 199920(4), 519-527.

[30] Griffiths, HR; Mistry, P; Herbert, KE; Lunec, J. Molecular and cellular effects of ultraviolet light-induced genotoxicity. *Crit. Rev. Clin. Lab. Sci.,* 1998 35, 189–237.

[31] Ramaswamy, NT; Ronai, Z; Pelling, JC. Rapid activation of JNK1 in UV-B epidermal keratinocytes. *Oncogene,* 1998 16, 1501–1505.

[32] Fuchs, SY; Fried, VA; Ronai, Z. Stress activated protein kinases regulate protein stability. *Oncogene,* 1998 17, 1483–1490.

[33] Botelho, MC; Machado, JC; Brindley, PJ; Correia da Costa, JM. Targeting molecular signaling pathways of Schistosomahae-motobium infection in bladder cancer. *Virulence,* 2011 2(4), 267-279.

[34] Bornschein, J; Rokkas, T; Selgrad, M; Malfertheiner, P. Gastric cancer: clinical aspects, epidemiology and molecular background. *Helicobacter,* 2011 16(1), 45-52.

[35] Werness, BA; Levine, AJ; Howley, PM. Association of human papillomavirus types 16 and 18 E6 proteins with p53. *Science,* 1999 248, 76–79.

[36] Dyson, N; Howley, PM; Munger, K; Harlow, E. The human papilloma virus-16 E7 oncoprotein is able to bind to the retinoblastoma gene product. *Science,* 1989 243, 934–937.

[37] Slagle, BL; Zhou, YZ; Butel, JS. Hepatitis B virus integration event in human chromosome 17p near the p53 gene identifies the region of the chromosome commonly deleted in virus-positive hepatocellular carcinomas. *Cancer Res.,* 1991 51(1), 49-54.

[38] Matsubara, K; Tokino, T. Integration of hepatitis B virus DNA and its implications for hepatocarcinogenesis. *Mol. Biol. Med.,*1990 7(3), 243-260.

[39] Carrillo-Infante, C; Abbadessa, G; Bagella, L; Giordano, A. Viral infections as a cause of cancer (review). *Int. J. Oncol.,* 2007 30(6), 1521-1528.

[40] Hayes, RB. Genetic susceptibility and occupational cancer. *Med. Lav.,* 1995 86, 206–213.

[41] Huff, J. Chemicals associated with tumours of the kidney, urinary bladder and thyroid gland in laboratory rodents from 2000 US National Toxicology Program / National Cancer Institute bioassays for carcinogenicity. *IARC Sci. Pub.,* 1999 147, 211–225.

[42] Luch, A. Nature and nurture – lessons from chemical carcinogenesis. *Nat. Rev. Cancer,* 2005 5, 113–125.

[43] Yamagiwa, K; Ichikawa, K. Experimental study of the pathogenesis of carcinoma. *J. Cancer Res.,* 1918 3, 1–29.

[44] Beremblum, I; Shubik, P. The role of croton oil applications, associated with a single painting of a carcinogen, in tumor induction of the mouse's skin. *Br. J. Cancer,* 1947 1, 379–382.

[45] Foulds, L. The experimental study of tumor progression: a review. *Cancer Res.,* 1954 14, 327–339.

[46] Klaunig, JE; Kamendulis, LM; Xu, Y. Epigenetic mechanisms of chemical carcinogenesis. *Hum. Exp. Toxicol.,* 2000 19, 543–555.

[47] Gutiérrez, JB; Salsamendi, AL. Fundamientos de ciênciatoxicológica. *Diaz de Santos,* 2001, 155–177.

[48] Melnick, RL; Kohn, MC; Portier, CJ. Implications for risk assessment of suggested non-genotoxic mechanisms of chemical carcinogenesis. *Environ Health Perspect,* 1996 104, 123–134.

[49] Lutz, WK. A true threshold dose in chemical carcinogenesis cannot be defined for a population, irrespective of the mode of action. *Hum. Exp. Toxicol.,* 2000 19, 566–568.

[50] Park, BK; Kitteringham, NR; Maggs, JL; Pirmohamed, M; Williams, DP. The role of metabolic activation in drug-induced hepatotoxicity. *Annu. Rev. Pharmacol. Toxicol.,* 2005 45, 177–202.

[51] Rojas, M; Cascorbi, I; Alexandrov, K; Kriek, E; Auburtin, G; Mayer, L; Kopp-Schneider, A; Roots, I; Bartsch, H. Modulation of benzo[a]pyrenediolepoxide-DNA adduct levels in human white blood cells by CYP1A1, GSTM1 and GSTT1 polymorphism. *Carcinogenesis,* 2000 21, 35–41.

[52] Williams, GM. Mechanisms of chemical carcinogenesis and application to human cancer risk assessment. *Toxicology,* 2001 161, 3–10.

In: Alkylating Agents …
Editor: Yildiz Dincer

ISBN: 978-1-62618-487-9
© 2013 Nova Science Publishers, Inc.

Chapter II

Alkylating Agent Exposure and Its Relation with Cancer Risk

*Yildiz Dincer**

Istanbul University Cerrahpasa Medical Faculty,
Department of Biochemistry, Istanbul, Turkey

Abstract

Alkylating agents is an important class of chemical carcinogens. Some alkylating agents directly interact with DNA to form base adducts, whereas some of them are required metabolic activation by microsomal cytochrome p450 system in liver. O^6 methylguanine (O^6 MG) formed in cellular DNA by alkylating agents is a mutagenic lesion. O^6-methylguanine pairs with thymine during replication resulting in the conversion of guanine–cytosine to adenine–thymine pairs. Exposure of alkylating agents may be derived from smoked, salted fish-meat products, vegetable, cheese, beer, drinking water, tobacco, pesticides, various drugs and occupation. Alkylating agents can be synthesized endogenously in the body from their precursors found in diet. Endogenous nitrosation mainly occurs in stomach and colon. Consumption of cured/smoked meat and fish which contains precursors of alkylating agents, leads to the

* E-mail:yldz.dincer@gmail.com

formation of carcinogenic *N*-nitroso compounds in the acidic medium of stomach. Endogenous nitrosation can also occurs in various organs with chronic infection or inflammation. O^6 MG is repaired by O^6-methylguanine DNA methyltransferase (O^6-MGMT). This enzyme restores O^6-MG adducts by transferring the methyl group to itself at a specific cysteine residue. As a result of this automethylation O^6-MGMT become inactivated, and is not regenerated. De novo synthesis of new enzyme molecules is required for subsequent repair. Cells with low O^6-MGMT level are more susceptible to cytotoxic and mutagenic effects of alkylating agents. The O^6-alkylguanine-DNA adducts form interstrand cross-linking in DNA, block the replication and direct cell to apoptosis. Because of their lethal effect, alkylating agents are used in anti-cancer therapy. The presence of high levels of O^6-MGMT in tumors provides a powerful resistance to alkylating agent-based chemotherapy. The susceptibility of any tissue to mutagenic effect of alkylating agents is depend on the balance between the ability of the tissue to metabolise alkylating agents to carcinogenic intermediates, the extend of O^6-MG formation in cell, rate of repair by O^6-MGMT, and the extend of DNA replication which occurs when O^6-MG is present. This chapter highlights current knowledge on alkylating agents and their impacts in human body.

Introduction

Alkylating Agents

Alkylating agents are the chemical compounds that transfer alkyl groups to various molecules. Based on their chemical structure, they are classified as alkylsulfates, alkyl alkane sulfonates and N-nitroso compounds (NOCs) (Figure 1). NOCs have been classified as possible human carcinogens by the International Agency for Research on Cancer [1]. NOCs are divided into two major groups: N-nitrosamines and N-nitrosamides. Both groups of NOCs are characterized by a nitroso group bound to a nitrogen atom (-N-N=O). N-nitrosamines and N-nitrosamides are formed by the reaction of amines and amides, respectively, with nitrosating agents. Nitrosating agents are nitrous acid, nitrous acidium ion and nitrous anhydride that are derived from nitrite (NO_2).

$NO_2^- + H^+ \rightleftharpoons HNO_2$ (Nitrous acid) $HNO_2 + H^+ \rightleftharpoons (H_2NO_2)^+$ (nitrous acidium ion)

$2HNO_2 \rightleftharpoons N_2O_3 + H_2O$ (Nitrous anhydride)

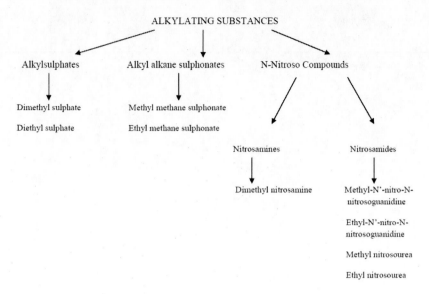

Figure 1. Groups of the alkylating substances.

N-nitrosamines are formed by nitrosation of secondary amines including dialkyl, alkylaryl groups. N-nitrosamides are formed by nitrosation of amides such as N-alkylamides, N-alkylureas and N-alkylcarbamates [2, 3].

$$RR'NH + N_2O_3 \rightleftharpoons RR'NNO + HNO_2 \text{ (Nitrosamines)}$$

$$RNHCOR' + (H_2NO_2)^+ \rightleftharpoons RN(NO)COR' + H_2O + H^+ \text{ (Nitrosamides)}$$

Although NOCs are environmental carcinogens, are also produced enzymatically in vivo. NOCs may be formed endogenously in the stomach and colon by the reactions between dietary nitrite and amines or amides. N-nitrosamides react DNA directly and lead to DNA adducts. Mechanism of DNA alkylation by N-nitroso compounds is shown in the Figure 2. N-nitrosamines are inactive and undergo activation in the human body to act as carcinogen. Although various organs and cells have been shown to be capable of carrying out metabolic activation, it mainly happens in liver. The human cytochrome P450 iso-enzymes, CYP1A2, CYP2A3, CYP2E1 and CYP2D6 bioactivate nitrosamines by a C-hydroxylation in the *N*-alkyl groups [4]. This results in the formation of aldehydes and *N*-nitrosomonoalkylamine intermediates.

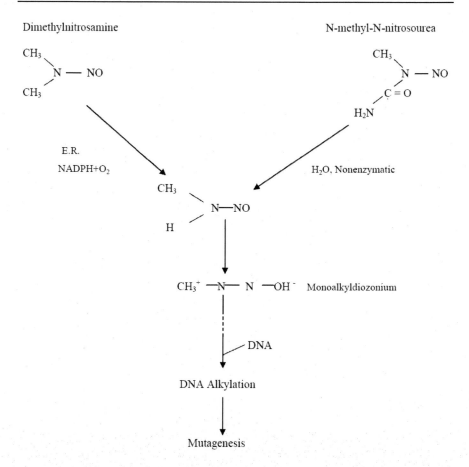

Figure 2. Mechanism of DNA alkylation by N-nitroso compounds.

The *N*-nitroso-monoalkylamines decompose to alkyldiazohydroxides, alkyldiazonium ions and ultimately into alkylcarbonium ions. Alkylcarbonium ions are electrophilic, unstable intermediate products that attack nucleophilic sites of DNA and form premutagenic DNA adducts. Carcinogenic potential of direct alkylating agents is higher than those of alkylating agents required metabolic activation.

Initially, carcinogenic potential of N-nitrosodiemthylamine in rats was demonstrated in 1956 [5]. After that, carcinogenic properties of NOCs was extensively investigated in laboratory animals. NOCs were shown to induce tumor development in liver, lung, nasopharynx, esophagus, stomach, pancreas, urinary bladder and bone. It was determined that N-nitrosamines are highly organotropic, animal species specific and may induce tumors in various organs independent of the route of administration. N-nitrosamides was determined to induce tumor development in various organs but especially in nervous system. Studies show that human and rodent liver metabolize nitrosamines in a similar manner, and DNA adducts formed in animals are similar to those detected in human studies. [2, 6, 7].

DNA Alkylation by N-Nitroso Compounds

NOCs exert their carcinogenic effects by forming mutagenic alkyl-DNA lesions. NOCs can react with various sites on DNA. Especially, nitrogen and oxygen atoms on the rings of purines and pyrimidines, and oxygen atoms of the phosphate groups which are not involved in 5'-3' phosphodiester bonds are major targets for DNA alkylation. The relative proportion of alkylation at the N and O atoms of purines and pyrimidines depends on the kind of alkylating agents. Alkylating agents cause non-coding and miscoding lesions. Non-coding lesions may be lethal. They arise either through depurination and depyrimidination which in turn lead strand breaks or by elimination of the ability of a base to serve as template during DNA replication. Bulky lesions cause both the depurination and inhibition of base pairing sterically. Miscoding lesions are mutagenic. They arise from which altered pattern of hydrogen bond donor and acceptor groups on the bases either by changing their protonation or by locking-in transformation to tautomeric structure. All lesions may induce DNA repair mechanisms. Enhanced base excision repair and nucleotide excision repair can lead to an increase in frequency of apurinic/apyrimidinic sites that can also contribute to mutations and cell death. DNA replication block derived from lesions can also be overcome by the induction of SOS repair. The SOS response is an inducible DNA repair system upon treatment of DNA with a damaging agent. Induction of the SOS response involves more than forty independent SOS genes. SOS bypass polymerases are the enzymes bypassing the damaged base during the replication. Although SOS response is described in many bacterial species, is not determined in eukaryotic cells. However, all species contain some SOS-like proteins taking part in DNA repair that exhibit amino acid homology and enzymatic activities related to those found in E. coli [8].

Various alkyl-DNA adducts are generated when DNA is treated with an alkylating agent in vitro. There are substantial evidence that O^6-methylguanine is the major responsible lesion for alkylating agent-mediated carcinogenesis.

O^6-methylguanine may be formed by at least three different mechanisms; direct alkylation of G.C base pairs in double stranded DNA, alkylation of guanine in single stranded DNA nearby replication forks, and alkylation of guanine in the nucleoside triphosphate pool followed by incorporation of O^6-methyl deoxyguanosine triphosphate during DNA replication. O^6-methylguanine mispairs mainly with T instead of C to give G.C $\rightarrow$ A.T mutation (Figure 3). Beyond causing mutation, O^6-methylguanine can lead the epigenetic changes in mammalian cells. O^6-methylguanine can inhibit the formation of 5-methylcytosine within the CpG dinucleotide by interfering with the binding of DNA methyltransferases. This inhibition in natural methylation can cause to DNA hypomethylation. In addition, the pairing of O^6-methylguanine with thymine can also lead to genome hypomethylation. Recent studies have suggested that O^6-methylguanine in DNA leads misincorporation of uridine by RNA polymerases and produces altered proteins at the transcriptional level. [9-11].

O^4-methylthymine is one of the mutagenic lesions formed concurrently with O^6- methylguanine but is formed at a much lower level than it. O^4-methylthymine is determined at a level 126 times lower than that of O^6-methylguanine in calf thymus DNA treated with methylnitrosourea.

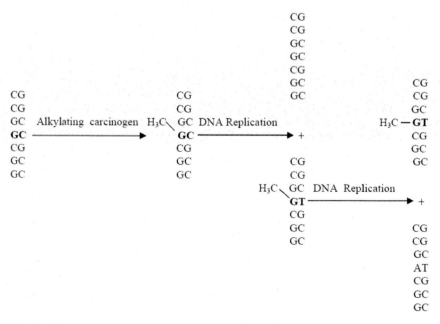

Figure 3. O^6-methylguanine -mediated mutagenesis.

However, it is very mutagenic. O^4-methylthymine pairs with G to cause A.T → G.C mutation.

N^3 *methyladenine* can be formed on DNA by alkylating agents as well as by S-adenosylmethionine. N^3 methyladenine leads to depurination/depyrimidination and formation of apurinic/apyrimidinic sites. It is able to block replication and because of this feature it is a lethal lesion rather than become mutagenic. N^3 methyladenine is suggested to cause p53 induction, S phase arrest, sister chromatid exchange, chromosome aberrations and apoptosis in mammalian cells [12].

N^1 *methyladenine*, N^1-*ethyladenine*, N^1 *methylguanine and* N^3 *methylguanine* are minor lesions and both of them block the DNA replication.

N^7 *methylguanine and* N^7 *methyladenine* are lethal lesions. The N^7 atom of guanine has the highest negative electrostatic potential of all the other atoms in the DNA bases. This feature makes it the most susceptible site to attacks of alkylating agents. N^7 methylguanine is the most abundant lesion in alkylated DNA. N^7 methyladenine is a minor lesion. Both N^7 methylguanine and N^7 methyladenine facilitate depurination and formation of apurinic sites and lead to blockage of replication. In addition, both of them have their imidazole ring-opened forms. Hydrolysis of the imidazole ring of N^7 methylguanine forms 2,6 diamino -4-hydroxy- 5N-methyl-formamidopyrimidine (Fapy-7MeG). This not mutagenic but a lethal lesion. Fapy-7MeG blocks DNA chain elongation. Imidazole ring-opened form of N^7 methyladenine (Fapy-7MeA) is a mutagenic lesion causing to A → G transition [13]. As respect with the fact that N^7 methyladenine appears at a very low level in alkylated DNA, its mutagenity is not considered very important for alkylating agent-mediated carcinogenesis.

N^8-*methylguanine* is a less-studied DNA alkylation damage. It is derived from attack of methyl radicals generated by oxidation of methylhydrazine and dimethylhydrazine. N^8-methylguanine can also be formed by genotoxic agents such as tert-butylhydroperoxide, diazoquinones and arenediazonium ions. It blocks the replication in mammalian cells, and is a weakly mutagenic lesion. N^8-methylguanine can lead to G → C transversion. N^8-methylguanine adducts may be a prime target for future investigations. Because, it is found to have a role in the regulation of DNA supercoiling. In addition, N^8-methylguanine is proposed as a chemical modification to stabilize quadruplex structures of G-rich sequences in DNA which are suggested to take part in both repression of transcription at the promoter of c-myc oncogene and in telomeric DNA stability [13, 14].

N^3 *methylcytosine and* N^3-*ethylcytosine* are likely to be lethal. N^3 methylcytosine blocks replication. Various investigations show that mutagenicity and cytotoxicity of N^3 methylcytosine are overcome by repair enzymes, AlkB protein and SOS bypass polymerases, respectively. If a cell has no AlkB and uninduced SOS bypass polymerases, N^3 methylcytosine and N^3-ethylcytosine exhibit 30% mutagenicity by causing C → T and C → A mutations. [13, 15-17].

N^3-methyltymine is a replication blocking lesion. It is very weak substrate for AlkB and can be just slightly overcome by SOS bypass polymerases.

Methyl phosphotriesters are the lesions formed by alkylating agents at the oxygen atoms of the phosphate internucleotide linkages. In vitro studies show that 17% of the total alkylation occurs on the DNA sugar-phosphate backbone. This lesion facilitates the cleavage of the backbone. The repair of methyl phosphotriesters in mammalian DNA apparently does not happen readily. Removal of methyl group was barely detected in mouse tissues. Cell culture extracts prepared from human liver or other human cells did not exhibit an effective repair activity against substrates containing phosphotriesters. It is suggested that methyl phosphotriesters may not have lethal lesions; their role seems to become a chemosensory for detection of methylation damage and induction of adaptive response in E. Coli, but their role in eukaryotes is unknown [18].

Repair of Alkylated DNA

In general, repair of alkylation damage before the replication occurs by two different mechanisms; direct repair and excision repair. After the replication, mismatched O^6-methylguanine can also be repaired by mismatch repair system. Direct repair involves the direct transfer of the methyl group from guanine to the repair enzyme itself, thus causing to loss of enzymatic activity. The latter involves the removal of alkylated bases by excision repair systems. Repair mechanisms for alkylated DNA are essentially similar in both bacterial and mammalian cells. Repair systems which recognize damaged DNA seem to be universally distributed in living cells. Incidence of tumor development in animals treated with an alkylating agent correlates with inadequate repair of O^6-methylguanine adducts.

O^6-methylguanine is repaired in a single step by a methyltransferase, O^6-alkylguanine DNA alkyltransferase, which transfers the methyl (alkyl) group from guanine to one of its own cysteine residues in both bacterial and mammalian cells. Actually this transferase does not like a true enzyme.

Because transfer of the alkyl group inactivates the enzyme irreversibly. The enzyme acts only once, and its alkylated form is not able to attach to DNA. It detaches from DNA and goes degradation by ubiquitination pathway. De novo synthesis of new enzyme molecules is required for subsequent repair activity. The susceptibility of a cell to alkylation damage is directly related to the number of O^6-alkylguanine DNA alkyltransferase molecules in the cell. O^6-alkylguanine DNA alkyltransferase has a wide substrate specificity. The enzyme acting on O^6-methylguanine is also capable of repairing a variety of O-alkylgroups such as O^4-alkylthymine. Two different O^6-alkylguanine DNA alkyltransferases were determined in E. Coli; the constitutive Ogt protein and Ada protein.

Ada protein is highly inducible in response to alkylation damage as part of the adaptive response. This was revealed when E. coli treated with a low dose of alkylating agent acquired resistance to mutagenicity and cytotoxicity of following higher doses. Ada is a single 39 k-Da protein consisting of two domains. Each domain contains a cysteine acceptor. Carboxyl-terminal domain is responsible for the repair of O^6-alkylguanine and O^4-alkylthymine whereas amino-terminal domain is involved in the repair of methyl phosphotriesters. Transfer of alkyl groups to a specific cysteine residue triggers the adaptive response in E coli. Alkylation of Cys-38 of Ada allows the protein to act as a transcriptional activator for a number of genes encoding proteins that counteract alkylation damage, namely ada, AlkA, AlkB and aidB. Alkylation at Cys-38 decreases the overall negative charge on Ada. Reduction in the charge density leads to a 1000 fold increase in the interaction between Ada and negatively charged DNA [19].

Another DNA methyltransferase, Ogt protein, is constitutively expressed, is not induced. Ogt protein preferentially repairs O^4-alkylthymine and bulky adducts, does not repair methyl phosphotriesters. Mammalian cells have unique enzymatic activity, O^6-methylguanine DNA methyltransferase (O^6MGMT, EC 2.1.1.63), homolog to Ada and Ogt proteins. Mammalian O^6MGMT has the same action mechanism but is not inducible. Animal studies show that O^6MGMT level is only slightly increased in alkylating agent–treated rats by certain stimuli such as partial hepatectomy and glucocorticoids [20,21]. Mammalian O^6MGMT has a 35-fold higher affinity for O^6-methylguanine adducts than those for O^4-methylthymine. It is also effective in repairing larger lesions such as O^6-ethylguanine, O^6-benzylguanine and bulky lesions formed by tobacco-derived alkylating agents. The constitutive level of O^6MGMT varies considerably from tissue to tissue in mammals. In human, O^6MGMT activity in brain is determined as 10-fold lower than in liver, and significantly lower than in colon, esophagus and lung. Experimental studies based on alterations in O^6MGMT levels caused by genetic manipulations provide convincing evidence of its critical role after exposure to alkylating agents. Many studies suggest that the expression of O^6MGMT greatly reduces the cytotoxicity and mutagenicity of alkylating agents. Transgenic overexpression of O^6MGMT in various tissues such as thymus, liver, skin, colon and lung prevents the development of malignancies after exposure to alkylating agents. On the contrary, gene disruption leading to loss of O^6MGMT activity causes an increased incidence of malignancy in the liver, colon, thymus and lung in response to alkylating agents. Exposure to alkylating agents is main determinative factor for carcinogenesis. Because it is demonstrated that mice with the inactivated MGMT gene do not show an increased spontaneous tumor incidence in the absence of exposure to DNA-damaging agents. [22-29].

The toxicity of alkylating agents results from formation of apurinic/apyrimidinic sites, strand breaks, interstrand cross-links, and the recognition of O^6-methylguanine/thymine pair by the mismatch repair system. Recognition of the mispaired bases results to homologous recombination, sister chromatid exchanges, and cell death, either via triggering apoptotic pathways or via abortive repeated excision, and resynthesis of the thymine-containing daughter DNA strand [30]. The O^6-alkylguanine-DNA adducts cause to formation of crosslinks with the opposite cytosine residues, blocking DNA replication. Because of their lethal effect, alkylating agents (procarbazine, temozolomide, chloroethylating agents etc.) are used in anti-cancer therapy. Although O^6MGMT plays critical role in the prevention of mutations and tumor development, the presence of high levels of the enzyme in tumors provides a powerful resistance to alkylating agent-based chemotherapy. O^6MGMT activity was also linked to resistance to 6-thioguanine. 6-Thioguanine is readily methylated by S-adenosylmethionine to form S6-methylthioguanine after incorporation into DNA. S6-methylthioguanine is recognized by mismatch repair system leading to cell death. O^6MGMT binds to S6-methylthioguanine, but this adduct is a very poor substrate for the enzyme. It is thought that O^6MGMT impedes toxicity of S6-methylthioguanine by binding it, rather than direct adduct repair. [11, 31-33].

Mammalian O^6MGMT can be silenced by epigenetic changes. This silencing results an increased incidence of tumor development in healthy individuals but causes an increased response to alkylating agent-based chemotherapy in cancer patients. Some tumor cell lines lack O^6MGMT expression. These cells are often described as Mer‾ (methyl excision repair negative). The frequency of the Mer‾ status in various tumor cell lines is quite high. Gene hypermethylation is main responsible factor for silencing. Specific methylation at critic sites of O^6MGMT gene is an important factor in this inactivation. Promoter methylation of O^6MGMT may be increased by p53 and decreased by estradiol [34-38]. It was reported that O^6MGMT activity is lost frequently in association with hypermethylation of the promoter region in a wide spectrum of human tumors.

A number of genetic variants were determined in the human O^6MGMT gene. Because of the critical role of O^6MGMT in carcinogenesis and in response to alkylating agent-based chemotherapy, many studies attempted to correlate the polymorphisms in O^6MGMT gene with cancer incidence or response to cancer therapy. The results of these studies are contradictory and do not provide a consistent perspective [39]. Further large scale studies are needed.

In addition to the O^6MGMT, nucleotide excision repair pathway can also repair O^6methylguanine lesions, and mismatch repair system recognizes O^6MG.T base pair after replication and removes it. In fact, all the main mechanisms of DNA repair are involved in the repair of either primary alkylation products or secondary damages derived from those products such as a basic sites, strand breaks and interstrand cross-links. All DNA repair mechanisms are protective against cytotoxic and mutagenic effects of various damaging agents. O^6MGMT is suggested to be unique DNA repair enzyme enhancing DNA damage paradoxally. After exposure of E. coli to dibromomethane or 1,2-dibromoethane, an increased incidence of mutation and cell death was observed when human O^6MGMT, Ada-C, or Ogt were expressed. 1,2-dibromoethane reacts with the reactive cysteine in O^6MGMT to form a O^6MGMT-S-(2-bromoethyl) metabolite, which rearranges into unstable half mustard. DNA binding property of O^6MGMT causes this metabolite into close contact with DNA. It then reacts with guanine residues to form a covalent bond between O^6MGMT and DNA, thus N7-guanine adducts are formed. N7-guanine is the unique position which is fully characterized for DNA- O^6MGMT adducts, but multiple alternatives are possible for other adducts which could lead to toxicity and mutagenicity. This bulky lesion can be partly released by spontaneous depurination. Subsequent DNA repair reduces the size of DNA- O^6MGMT lesion which permits synthesis by bypass DNA polymerases causing mutations. Toxicity may arise when DNA-O^6MGMT lesions can not be bypassed by bypass DNA polymerases efficiently. All of the mutations were determined at G:C sites, G to T transversions which can be derived from apurinic sites after depurination of the adduct, and G to A transitions. [11, 40-43].

In addition to forming the DNA- O^6MGMT conjugation, exposure to agents which react readily with the active site cysteine results a direct loss of O^6MGMT activity. Aldehydes such as acrolein, formaldehyde, and acetaldehyde inactivate O^6MGMT by this way. Exposure to nitric oxide readily nitrosylates the active site cysteine residue of O^6MGMT. In the presence of S-nitrosylcysteine at Cys145 polyubiquitination of the O^6MGMT and its proteasomal degradation is induced. Conditions which increase the production of nitric oxide lead the loss of O^6MGMT. S-nitrosoglutathione reductase is the enzyme reversing the S-nitrosylation and may be effective in preventing such inactivation. Impaired repair of O^6-alkylguanine was demonstrated in mice lacking S-nitrosoglutathione reductase. In a recent investigation, protective effect of S-nitrosoglutathione on S-nitrosylation and subsequent proteasomal degradation of O^6MGMT was demonstrated in mice. Considering the fact that hepatocellular carcinoma is associated with increased expression of inducible nitric oxide synthase, and S-nitrosoglutathione reductase activity is frequently deficient in human hepatocellular carcinoma, it has been suggested that the incidence of hepatocellular carcinoma may be increased by defective O^6MGMT activity derived from low S-nitrosoglutathione reductase activity. [11, 44, 45].

Specific Mutations Induced by Alkylating Agents

Ras proto-oncogene can be transformed to an oncogene by single-point mutation within its coding sequences. In general, mutations in ras oncogenes are localized in codons 12, 13, 59 and 61. Alteration of codon 12, GGT, is the most common alteration. Mutationally activated K-ras in breast, lung, kidney, thyroid and colon tumors was demonstrated by early animal studies. The incidence of K-ras activation varies from one type of cancer to another. It was reported that the incidence of K-ras activation was the lowest in oesophagel cancer and the highest in colon cancer. G.C $\rightarrow$ A.T transitions are characteristic for alkylating agents. Determination of the presence of such characteristic ras mutations may be a possible fingerprint of nitroso compounds. Some animal studies were provided evidence. G.C $\rightarrow$ A.T transition in codon 12 of the ras gene was observed in rat mammary tumors induced by *N*-methyl-*N*nitrosourea, which indicates that activation of ras oncogene is a direct consequence of the interaction of the NOCs with DNA. *N*-

methyl-N-nitrosourea was reported to induce G.C → A.T transitions in codons 12 and 13 of K-ras in 30% of rat colon carcinomas. In human studies, G.C → A.T transitions at the second G of a GG pair in codon 12 or 13 of K-ras were commonly observed in colorectal cancer. However, on the contrary, ras mutations were not determined in human esophageal cancer in areas of exposure to N-nitrosomethylbenzylamine. This contradiction may be derived from differences in the repair activity of O^6MGMT in different human tissues. Repair rate of O^6methylguanine adducts is the major determinant for mutagenicity of NOCs. The link between O^6MGMT inactivation and K-ras transition mutations in human tumors was first suggested in 2000. O^6MGMT promoter hypermethylation was found to be an early event in human colorectal tumorigenesis linked to the appearance of G.C → A.T mutations in the K-ras. The association between O^6MGMT promoter methylation and K-ras mutations was supported by the subsequent studies in gastric and and gall bladder cancers. [34, 46-52].

O^6MGMT silencing is not likely to be limited to a relation with only K-ras mutations. The tumor suppressor p53 is the most commonly mutated gene in human cancers, especially in colorectal tumors. The main type of p53 mutations was observed as G:C → A: T transitions. Promoter hypermethylation of O^6MGMT was linked to the presence of G:C → A: T transition mutations in p53 gene in gliomas, colon, esophageal, and non-small-cell lung, carcinomas. [53-57].

Endogenous Formation of N-Nitroso Compounds

The G:C → A: T transition in codons 12 or 13 of K-ras is the common mutation in colorectal cancer. This brings to mind the presence of alkylating agents at a high concentration in the gastrointestinal tract. In vivo formation of N-nitrosotrimethylurea was detected in the pig stomach after administration of the trimethylurea and nitrite. N-nitrosoalkylurea formation and tumor development were demonstrated in the rats feeding with food which contains N-nitroso precursors methyl- and dimethylurea and drinking water containing nitrite. In order to examine the endogenous formation of NOCs in human gastrointestinal tract, foods were nitrosated in the laboratory under stimulated gastric conditions, combined with physiological concentrations of nitrite.

Results of these in vitro studies suggested that gastric conditions can cause to NOCs formation. [58-61].

As an evidence for endogenous production of NOCs, O^6methylguanine formation in human lymphocyte DNA was found in a large number of persons who don't exposure to environmental alkylating agents [62]. In the absence of any evidence for exogenous exposure to NOCs, presence of O^6methylguanine in DNA can be attributed to endogenous formation of NOCs. There are many possible sources of endogenous alkylation. S-Adenosylmethionine is a methyl-donor in biochemical reactions but is also a weak chemical methylating agent to induce mutations in DNA. It mainly generates 7-methylguanine and 3-methyladenine, but little O^6-methylguanine [63]. Nitrosated amines generate more effective mutagenic alkylating agents than S-Adenosylmethionine in vivo and are responsible for cancers developed in gastrointestinal tract. Two mechanisms of endogenous nitrosation were described; chemical nitrosation and bacterial nitrosation. Dietary amines and nitrates are the precursors of endogenously produced NOCs. Essential nutrients such as proteins and some metabolites such as urea are the main sources of amines. Nitrate and nitrite come from processed meats, vegetables and drinking water. Endogenous nitrosation occurs predominantly in the stomach. The chemical nitrosation happens at the low pH of the stomach between amine and amide precursors and nitrite which is generated from nitrate. Nitrates found in drinking water, fruits and vegetables are reduced to nitrite by bacterial nitrate reductase in saliva or in the achlorhydric stomach by bacteria. Nitrite can form nitrous acid (HNO_2) which reacts with amines to produce nitrosamines. Nitrosamines may exert their carcinogenic effects in stomach, or in other target organs via systemic circulation.

The second mechanism is the bacterial nitrosation in the stomach and colon, which occurs at a higher pH. Bacterial nitrosation occurs in achlorhydric stomach where a large numbers of bacteria are present. Amines and amides generated primarily by bacterial decarboxylation of amino acids can be N-nitrosated in the presence of nitrosating agents in the gut. In the anaerobic large bowel, dietary nitrate that reaches the colon is reduced to nitrite by dissimilatory nitrate metabolism of the colonic flora, and then nitrite acts as a nitrosating agent to form NOCs. In animals, N-nitrosation in the colon was demonstrated as dependent on the presence of gut flora.

Endogenous nitrosation not only occurs in stomach and colon but also in various organs with chronic infection or inflammation. During the infectious disease and at sites of chronic inflammation, nitric oxide (NO) is produced by phagocytic cells, especially by activated macrophages. NO is mainly synthesized in activated macrophages by inducible NO synthase which converts L-arginine into NO and L-citrillune. NO is the source of endogenously synthesized nitrite. Nitrosation of amines by activated macrophages is evidenced. Endogenous nitrosation may occur at various sites of the body, such as the oral cavity, stomach, colon, urinary bladder, and at other sites of infection or inflammation.

In vitro, nitrosation of amines and amides is accelerated by thiocyanates and organic acides, respectively. Thiocyanate and organic acids are natural constituents of the fruits and vegetables. Nitrosation of the precursors in foodstuffs by these mechanisms leads to the formation of NOCs, even after intake of levels that are considered to be normal daily amounts. Although variable, it is estimated that nearly 45%-75% of human exposure to NOCs is derived from in vivo formation [64].

Endogenously produced NOCs are suggested to be associated with an increased risk for gastrointestinal cancers. Colonic lumen contains a considerable amount of amines and amides, which are substrate for nitrosation. In addition, dietary nitrate is reduced to nitrite in the colon during nitrate metabolism of the colonic flora and is shown to increase faecal NOCs level. Endogenously produced NOCs in the colon is suggested to one explanation for the association between meat consumption and colon cancer in humans. Patients with chronic atrophic gastritis and pernicious anemia have an increased risk for gastric cancer, because achlorhydric stomach contains a large numbers of bacteria. As a matter of fact, gastric juice of such patients frequently contains higher nitrite and NOCs levels than that of healthy persons. Ulcerative colitis is one of the well-defined chronic inflammatory disease associated with endogenous formation of NOCs. Nitrite level in colonic dialysates is found to be higher in patients with ulcerative colitis than that in healthy cases. This nitrite is thought to produce from NO generated by inflammatory cells which are abundant in the lamina propria of active colitis. The another substrate for production of NOCs, primary or secondary amines, are produced by colonic bacteria, as well as lowered pH, a condition that occurs in patients with acute ulcerative colitis. The incidence of colorectal cancer development is significantly higher in patients with ulcerative colitis as compared to healthy persons, particularly if the inflammation is extensive and of long duration. It has been suggested that endogenous NOC formation constitutes the 10% risk of colon cancer in patients with ulcerative colitis. [3, 65].

In addition to gastrointestinal cancers, endogenously produced NOCs are suggested to be associated with an increased risk for urinary bladder cancer in bilharzia-infested individuals. Secondary bacterial infections of the urinary bladder are generally associated with bilharziasis. Nitrosamines can be formed because of increased conversion of nitrates to nitrites and the acidic pH of urine under such conditions, and may lead to tumor development in bladder urothelium. [66, 67] A number of inhibitors of N-nitrosation are determined to decrease the exposure of humans to NOCs. It is known that ascorbic acid, vitamin E and polyphenols strongly inhibit in vivo nitrosation [68]. Although, vitamin E acts as an inhibitor of in vivo nitrosation, it is less effective. These inhibitors are natural compounds found in fruits, vegetables, green tea and grains. Nitrate is present at high levels in some vegetables, however, the presence of nitrosation inhibitors in vegetables may limit in vivo NOCs formation. It is demonstrated that after four weeks of treatment of ascorbic acid, a significant decrease is determined in NOCs concentration of gastric juice of hypochlorhydric individuals. Formation and urinary excretion of NOCs were shown to blocked by consumption of 2–5 g of tea daily in humans, and this effect was attributed the presence of polyphenols in tea [69]. According to these data, inhibition of endogenous NOC production by vitamin C and polyphenols may account for reduction of gastric cancer. As for bacterial nitrosation, blocking effect of garlic on the growth of nitrate reducing bacteria and on the production of nitrite; the inhibitor effect of an oral antiseptic mouthwash solution containing chlorhexidine on the nitrate–nitrite conversion in the oral cavity were examined. From these studies, it can be concluded that nitrosation inhibitors can reduce the formation of NOCs in stomach; however, it is not clear what the effect of these nitrosation inhibitors is on the NOCs exposure in the colon [4].

Exogenous Exposure to N-Nitroso Compounds

Humans are exposed to preform NOCs in the environment through ingestion or inhalation. Human exposure to N-nitroso compounds and their precursors, nitrates and nitrites, occurs through exogenous sources such as diet, drinking water, smoking, occupation, alkylating drugs or environmental exposures including pharmaceutical products, cosmetics, indoor and outdoor air.

Diet

Meats

Nutrition has been implicated in cancer etiology for a long time. Diet is the major source of exposure to NOCs and their precursors in humans. Dietary NOCs intake is determined by the type and amount of consumed foods which include alkylating agents and their precursors. Many nitrosatable substances, precursors of NOCs, are available in foods which can produce both amines and amides under acidic conditions of stomach following ingestion. Precursors of NOCs are present in foods that contain nitrite or have been exposed to nitrogen oxides, such as nitrite-cured and smoked meat, fish, cheese and vegetable. Nitrates and nitrites have been used since ancient times as preserving and curing substances for meats. Nitrites inhibit the growth of spore-forming bacteria in foods which may cause fatal food poisoning. They are also used to add color and flavor to meats. In the absence of nitrites meat darkens in colour. Because the Fe^{2+}-haem in myoglobin is oxidized to give dull-red metmyoglobin. NO binds to myoglobin to give a red complex which decreases oxidation. Despite these advantages, nitrite can react with amines to generate nitrosamines in acidic medium of stomach. Processed meats are not only a source of nitrate and nitrite, but also a source of amines and amides, which are other precursors of NOCs. Therefore, ingestion of nitrate or nitrite from processed meats should cause much more exposure to NOCs than plant-based foods.

Processed meat includes ham, sausage, bacon, liverwurst, salami, tinned and corned meat. It is generally made from beef or pork, but various specific meat products and some vegetables are processed by traditional methods all over the world. The aim of the processing is to preserve the food and to improve its quality, flavor and color. Processing methods are curing, drying and smoking.

The curing process is the addition of the salt, sugar and nitrate/nitrite. Nitrite inhibits the growth of clostridium botulinum spores and keeps the bright pink-red colour of meat by binding to heme iron as mentioned above. Salt inhibits the bacterial growth by diffusing into the muscle and reducing the water activity in it, furthermore improves the taste of meat [70]. Curing can be performed with dry salt, in a brine tank or by injection. In the dry salting, meat is placed on stack of salt, rubbed with a large amount of mixture of salt, sugar and sodium nitrate, and then kept at the low temperature until the center of the meat piece is salted enough to prevent bacterial activity. In the tank curing, meat pieces are placed in water saturated with salt which also includes sugar and nitrite. This is a faster method than dry curing. In order to accelerate the diffusion rate of curing agents into meat, multi-needle injection systems were developed for commercial businesses.

Smoking or drying of food is made by exposing food to smoke from incomplete wood pyrolysis or warm air, respectively. In the drying at the warm air process, air contains higher percentage of nitrogen than normal air to avoid the oxidation of fatty acids in the meat. This method prevents the rancidity but nitrogen acts as a potential nitrosating agents to amines or amides. Smoking gives meat a brown colour, changes its flavor and inhibits bacterial growth in the meat. Because it contains acetic acid, phenols and aldehydes. Beyond alkylating agents, smoke may include polycyclic aromatic hydrocarbons which is an another class of carcinogens. Smoking process can be performed without contamination of polycyclic aromatic hydrocarbons by immersing meat cuts into a smoke solution that provides smoke flavor [70].

Human studies show that consumption of red meat increases the intestinal N-nitrosation and fecal NOCs excretion. Upon this finding attentions were focused on heme, and heme was suggested as a stimulator of endogenous NOC formation in the gastrointestinal tract. Two mechanisms were suggested as possible pathways for this impact of heme. Firstly, N-nitrosomyoglobin which is an alkylating agent may be formed by the reaction between nitrite and myoglobin. Secondly, NO may react directly with myoglobin to form NOCs. A study carried on ileostomists demonstrated that heme can facilitates the NOCs formation in the absence of colonic flora in the upper gastrointestinal tract. In the ileostomists fed with fresh red meat or processed meat, endogenous NOCs excretion in the ileostomy output was found to be 4-fold or 6.5 fold increased, respectively. [71-74].

Increased consumption of red and processed meat is determined to be associated with an increased risk of certain types of cancer. Especially, the association between consumption of red/processed meat and risk of colorectal cancer, gastric cancer and brain tumors are extensively investigated. Epidemiologic studies show that countries where people eat more red meat are also countries where incidence of colorectal cancer is high [75]. Fecal NOCs level in individuals who are fed with a high red meat diet is higher. According to three meta-analyses taking all previous studies into account; a high fresh red meat (beef, veal, pork, mutton, lamb, offal) consumption is associated with a moderate and significantly increased colorectal cancer risk whereas processed meat (sausages, meat burgers, ham, Bacon, salami, nitrite-treated meats) consumption is associated with increased risk , the risk associated with intake of one gram processed meat is two to ten times higher than the risk associated with the intake of one gram of fresh red meat [76-78]. Subsequent few studies also supported the results of meta-analyses although individual studies were seldom significant. In a study performed in the U.S.A., higher colorectal cancer risk for people who did not reduce their consumption of red meat and processed meat, especially pork and ham, after the age of 30 years was reported [79]. Although NOCs are carcinogenic in laboratory animals and leads to ras mutations which are frequently identified in colon tumors, it was found in a study that processed meat intake caused to increased fecal excretion of NOCs but did not initiate and promote the aberrant crypt foci [80]. This contradiction may be explained by the fact that, estimation of colorectal cancer risk with fresh/processed meat intake may be influenced by other dietary nutrients. Fats, bile acids, polycyclic aromatic hydrocarbons and heterocyclic amines are also suspected factors for colorectal cancer. In addition, differences in bioactivation process may be determinative. As a common finding of major studies, increased risk of colorectal cancer by high meat diet, processed or not, declines with the higher consumption of fiber and micronutrients such as polyphenols, vitamin C, and vitamin E which are referred as nitrosation inhibitors.

Processed seafoods are also a high source of NOCs. Incidence of gastro-esophageal cancers is very high in some regions of Asia. Frequent consumption of aged and smoked fish products and vegetables is suspected to be related to these cancers. Further evidence supporting this hypothesis came from Finland where smoked and processed fish is frequently consumed. In a large scale Finland cohort N-nitrosodimethlyamine ingestion from smoked and salted fish was found to be associated with colorectal cancer risk [81].

There are many environmental toxins suspected for contributing to development of brain tumors. Among these, NOCs are extensively investigated over the last three decades. Brain tumors are the most common solid tumors in children. The occurrence of childhood brain tumor is highest in children under five years of age. Carcinogenic compounds are capable of crossing the placental barrier, entering the fetal circulation and interacting with DNA in the developing fetus. Rapid cell growth and proliferation in fetus give the opportunity for mutagenic changes potentially leading to tumor formation. Animal studies demonstrate that fetal brain is less able to efficiently repair the alkylated DNA, and is more vulnerable than other organs to transplacental exposure to carcinogens. Induction of brain tumors by N-alkylnitrosoureas in the offspring of various animals are demonstrated by early studies. By extrapolating the animal data to humans association between NOCs exposure and brain cancers is plausible. In many of epidemiologic studies including complete dietary surveys, maternal consumption of cured meats is the factor most closely related to increased risk of childhood brain tumor [82-84]. On the other hand, no significant increased glioma risk with increased intake of processed or red meat, nitrite or nitrate are also reported. [82-88].

Nitrate and nitrite use in meat products is subject to limits put forth in Food and Drug Administration (FDA) and US Department of Agriculture (USDA) regulations. These regulations can be found in the Code of Federal Regulations (CFR) (21CFR 170.60, 172.170, and 172.175 for FDA and 9CFR 318.7 for USDA regulations respectively). On the basis of the association with cancer risk, the American Institute for Cancer Research's Food, Nutrition, Physical Activity, and the Prevention of Cancer: a Global Perspective includes the following suggestion 'Limit consumption of red meats and avoid processed meats'.

Consumption of 500 g weekly of red meat is indicated as threshold limit quantity for cancer risk. However, a safe consumption level for processed meat is not determined; based on a meta-analysis of cohort studies, colon cancer risk increases with any consumption of processed meats. [89, 90].

Vegetables

Nitrate and nitrite are natural components of plants. They are found at high concentrations in leafy vegetables, such as spinach, lettuce, cabbage and some root vegetables such as carrot and beet. Nitrate intake from plant sources depends on the type and amount of the consumed vegetable and nitrate level in the vegetable.

Nitrate content of a vegetable is determined by the factors such as genotype of vegetable, soil conditions, growth conditions, and storage and transport conditions after harvesting. Therefore, nitrate content of a vegetable may change in a large scale. Nitrate and nitrite contents of some vegetables are given in Table 1. In addition to fresh vegetables, smoked vegetables are frequently consumed in some areas of Asia. This habit increases the cancer risk. The association between increased risk of colon cancer and high intake of preserved meat and vegetable is demonstrated in Shangai. [91, 92]

Many of the vegetables contain vitamin C, vitamin E and polyphenols which are inhibitors of endogenous nitrosation. When nitrate is consumed as part of a normal diet containing vegetables, nitrosation inhibitors are also concomitantly consumed. Therefore, dietary nitrate may not give rise to substantial formation of NOCs.

Table 1. Nitrate and nitrite concentrations of some vegetables[a]

Vegetable types and varieties	Nitrite			Nitrate		
	mg/100 g fresh weight			mg/100 g fresh weight		
Root vegetables						
Carrot	0.002-0.023			92-195		
Mustard leaf	0.012-0.064			70-95		
Green vegetables						
Lettuce	0.008-0.215			12.3-267.8		
Spinach	0-0.073			23.9-387.2		
Cabbage						
Chinese cabbage	0-0.065			42.9-161.0		
Bok choy	0.009-0.242			102.3-309.8		
Cabbage	0-0.041			25.9-125.0		
Cole	0.364-0.535			76.6-136.5		
Melon						
Wax gourd	0.001-0.006			35.8-68.0		
Cucumber	0-0.011			1.2-14.3		
Nightshade						
Eggplant	0.007-0.049			25.0-42.2		

[a] Data from reference 139.

Drinking Water

Nitrate is an environmental contaminant which results from the use of nitrogen fertilizers in agricultural areas and from human and animal waste via sewage disposal systems. Nitrogen fertilizer use increased over five-fold in industrialized countries. Nitrate is the final breakdown product of nitrogen fertilizers. It accumulates in ground water under agricultural areas. Nitrate levels can also be high in streams and rivers due to runoff of excess nitrogen fertilizer from agricultural fields. High exposure to nitrate may inhibit the oxygen-carrying capacity of the blood by causing methemoglobinemia in infants. The permissible nitrate content of drinking water was declared as 50 mg nitrate/L for European Union and 44 mg nitrate/L for U.SA. by the World Health Organisation in 1970. The United States Environmental Protection Agency limited the maximum contaminant level of nitrate as 10 mg/L nitrate–nitrogen (i.e., the total amount of nitrogen in the nitrate) for public water supplies. This level was set to protect against methemoglobinemia. [93-96] However, drinking water can be a major source of nitrate intake which leads to endogenous formation of NOCs when its concentration is above the maximum contaminant level.

Endogenous nitrosation is measured by excretion of N-nitroso compounds such as N-nitrosoproline or *N*-nitrosodi-methylamine. In humans, nitrate levels in drinking water were associated with excreted nitrate and N-nitrosoproline levels in urine, and nitrate administration via drinking water was found to be directly related to concentration of total NOCs in feces. In another study, a 200% increase in excretion of the *N*-nitrosodi-methylamine in the urine was determined after ingestion of nitrate in drinking water at the acceptable daily intake level in combination with fish meal rich in amines as nitrosatable precursors. A significant correlation was also established between nitrate in drinking water and excretion of *N*-nitrosodi-methylamine.[97-100] Most epidemiologic studies investigating the relation between nitrate concentration of drinking water and cancer were ecologic in design, linking incidence or mortality rates to drinking water nitrate concentrations for large groups at the town or county level. Although most epidemiologic studies were concurrent with the time period of cancer incidence or mortality, their results were contradictory. In Colombia and Italy, high levels of nitrate in well water were determined to be associated with an increased risk of gastric cancer, as the first time in 1976 and 1984 respectively. These results demonstrate a contribution of drinking water to overall nitrosation and show increased cancer risk. On the other hand, in the ecologic studies carried out in Valencia-Spain and Ontario-Canada no association was determined between bladder cancer rates and nitrate levels in water supplies. In agreement with these studies, in Slovakia and Germany no association was found between kidney cancer incidence and nitrate levels of public supply that were slightly above the acceptable level. In a cohort study including older women in Iowa no association was determined between kidney cancer risk and higher average nitrate exposures from public water over about 30 years. In Iowa, a direct association was not established between colorectal cancer risk and nitrate level in public water supplies and it was suggested that any increased risk of colon cancer associated with nitrate in public water supplies might occur only among susceptible subpopulations such as those with a history of inflammatory bowel disease. [94, 101-107].

In 1991, a case-control study in Germany determined an association between risk of gastric cancer and private well water use [108]. Groundwater is used as drinking water by nearly 90% of the people who are living in countryside of United States and many rural residents have private wells. Private wells often have higher nitrate levels than public supplies because they are often more shallow than public wells, and may not be well constructed to prevent leakages form surroundings. They are not regulated by the United States Environmental Protection Agency under the Safe Drinking Water Act.

According to a survey of private well-water users in Iowa, 35% of wells less than 50 feet deep have nitrate levels higher than the maximum contaminant level. In a cohort study in Iowa, in 2001, a 2.8-fold elevated risk of bladder cancer was found among those with public water supply nitrate levels above 2.5 mg/liter nitrate-nitrogen. They also determined no significant exposure-response association for leukemia, melanoma, non-Hodgkin lymphoma, and cancers of pancreas and lung. However, two years later, it was reported that long-term exposure to nitrate in drinking water at the level of 5.5 mg/liter nitrate-nitrogen (90th percentile) was not associated with risk of bladder cancer in Iowa. [107, 109, 110].

Taken together, making interpretation is highly difficult. Differences in the results of studies may be explained by the limitations including the study design, use of mortality data, and difficulties in the elimination of other confounding factors. Estimating NOCs formation via nitrate ingestion with drinking water requires a very detailed information on dietary (red and processed meat, vegetables, nitrosatable drugs, amount of nitrosation inhibitors in diet) and drinking water sources of nitrate, and medical conditions which may increase nitrosation (chronic infectious and inflammatory diseases). In addition, as respect with the fact that some NOCs are required metabolic activation to act as a carcinogen, it is important to examine the roles of polymorphisms in the genes involved in the bioactivation of NOCs.

Preformed nitrosamines are found in beer and to a lesser extent, distilled spirits. Beer contains volatile nitrosamines because of the malting process and is considered an important source of nitrosamines. N-nitrosodimethylamine in beer was discovered first time in 1980 as a result of comprehensive survey of nitrosamines in foods and beverages in Germany. The highest N-nitrosodimethylamine levels were measured in dark and smoky beer which have a high content of malt. The origin of N-nitrosodimethylamine was suggested as alkaloids, hordenine and gramine, available in barley. These alkoloids are derivatives of dimethylamine and are readily nitrosated by nitric oxides present in the flue gases from the burning of the fuel used to heat the malt and allowed to come in contact with it. After the discovery of this fact, nitrosamine level in beer was reduced to acceptable level (5ppm) by sequestering the malt from the gases. N-nitrosodimethylamine arising from the barley malt is also present in various kinds of whisky. However whisky has a lower cancer risk. Because it has a lower N-nitrosodimethylamine content than in beer, and whisky is consumed by people in smaller amounts than beer. It should be noted that although regulations in beer manufacture reduced the level of nitrosamines in beer, large amount of beer consumption every day leads to ingestion of a considerably amount of nitrosamine. On the other hand, ethanol was also demonstrated in several animal studies to suppress hepatic clearance of nitrosamines which in turn increases internal exposure. In addition, acetaldehyde produced during the metabolism of ethanol was discovered to interfere with DNA repair by directly inhibiting O^6MGMT. [111-115].

Table 2. High food sources of N-nitroso compounds [a]

Compound	High source foods
N-nitrosodimethylamine	Beer, sausage, cured meats
N-nitrosodiethylamine	Sausage, cheese
N-nitrosopyrrolidine	Fried bacon, sausage, ham
N-nitrosopiperidine	Bologna, sausage
N-nitrosarcosine	Cured meats
N-nitrosoproline	Fried bacon, cured meats
N-nitrosotioazolidine-4-carboxylic acid	Smoked meats
N-nitrososo-2-hydroxymethylthiazolidine-4-carboxylic acid	Smoked meats
Nitrate (precursor of nitrosating agent)	Vegetables, grains
Nitrite (nitrosating agent)	Additive to meats, other foods
Amines (become nitrosated)	Protein foods
Amides (become nitrosated)	Protein foods

[a]Adapted from reference 141.

In 2006, a working group convened by the International Agency for Research on Cancer (IARC) concluded that ingested nitrate or nitrite under conditions that result in endogenous formation of NOCs was probably carcinogenic to humans (Group 2A). It should also be taken into consideration that NOCs were demonstrated to cause cancer in every animal species that have been tested. It is unlikely that humans are not affected. [93, 116, 117] According to N-nitroso database established by Stuff [91] N-nitroso content of food items ranges from <0.01 µg/100 g. to 142 µg/100 g. and the richest sources are sausage, smoked meats, bacon, and luncheon meats. NOCs present in high food sources are shown in the Table 2.

Smoking

Inhalatory exposure to tobacco smoke probably represents the main source of exogenous exposure to NOCs for humans. Cigarette smoking has been shown to be significantly associated with alkylation damage. Tobacco smoke contains volatile and non-volatile nitrosamines. They occur at high concentrations in tobacco smoke and at even higher concentrations in snuff and chewing tobacco which are used in some parts of world. Volatile nitrosamines contribute the cancer risk associated with passive exposure to smoke. Among the known tobacco-specific nitrosamines, the most carcinogenic in laboratory animals are 4-(methylnitrosamino)-1-(3-pyridyl)-1-butanone (NNK), 4-(methylnitrosamino)-1-(3-pyridyl)-1-butanol (NNAL), and *N*-nitrosonornicotine (NNN). NNAL is a metabolite of NNK. All are required metabolic activation to act as a carcinogen. In experimental studies in animals and also in human tissues in vitro, NNK, NNAL and NNN were shown to be readily converted to electrophilic compounds which can react with DNA. In order to monitor environmental exposure to tobacco-specific nitrosamines, several potential biomarkers have been assessed. Among these NNAL seems best suited biomarker. NNAL and its glucuronides are metabolites of NNK and give specific and reliable quantitative information on exposure to tobacco smoke. In animal studies, the principle organs affected by smoke-specific nitrosamines are trachea, nasal cavity, lung and oesophagus which are the major target sites at cancer risk in humans who smoke. NNK plays a major role in lung carcinogenesis, it systemically induces tumors of the lung in rats, mice, and hamsters. As previously reported in mouse and rat studies, NNK exposure not only leads to gene mutation, but also induces epigenetic changes including hypermethylation of multiple tumor suppressor gene promoters in liver or lung tumors. In a recent study it has been shown that NNK induces DNA methyltransferase 1 nuclear accumulation and hypermethylation of the promoters of tumor suppressor genes which may give rise to carcinogenesis. This finding provides an evidence for the link between tobacco smoking and lung cancer. [118-124].

Some of the tobacco-specific nitrosamines may also be formed by endogenous nitrosation of tobacco alkaloids. Myosmine, a tobacco alkaloid, is present in a variety of foods, including several fruits, vegetables and even milk, and it is easily nitrosated to NOCs [125, 126].

Occupation

Nearly all industries which involve the production and/or usage of amines have a related nitrosamine problem. In industries such as rubber and tyre manufacture, leather tanning and metal working, relatively high concentrations of volatile NOCs are detected frequently in the grinding fluids and in surrounding air. In metal industry, N-nitrosodiethanolamine are found in cutting fluids which contain diethanolamine and nitrite as anticorrosive agents.

Cutting oil mist can be inhaled, penetrate the skin, or contaminate other products. N-nitrosodiethanolamine was monitored in the urine of exposed workers, and this NOC was detected in some cosmetic products. N-nitrosodimethylamine formation was detected in leather tanning industry, and this was attributed to chemicals used in the depilation process. Rubber manufacturing involves many agents which are well defined carcinogens and a considerable exposure to nitrosamines occurs during manufacturing. A positive association between occupational nitrosamine exposure and having detectable O^6-methylguanine adducts in peripheral blood has been found in rubber industry workers. [7, 118, 127].

Beyond the industrial environment, contact with cosmetics, rubber products, pesticides and packaging materials may subject to contamination by low concentrations of NOCs. This contamination may be derived from the use of contaminated starting materials or from the production of NOCs during manufacturing. Many pesticides contain amine or amide groups which can react with nitrite and thus are potential precursors for NOCs in vivo. More than 300 pesticide formulations include nitrosamines and are able to react with nitrite. Nitrosamine contamination was detected in many pesticides commonly used in agriculture. The contamination may occur either in the manufacturing process or through the reaction of amine containing pesticides with nitrite that was used as a preservative or anticorrosive. Workers employed in pesticide production, farmers and other pesticide applicators may be under the risk of exposure. Carcinogenicity of the different pesticides differs depending on ability of each pesticide to form NOCs.

Exposure to nitrosatable pesticides or to pesticides contaminated with nitrosamines was suggested as a possible cause of the higher rates of brain cancer among farmers. N-nitrosoureas were determined to be strongest potent neurocarcinogens in early animal studies. In cohort studies, in agreement with animal studies, licensed pesticide users in Italy and golf course superintendents in the USA were found to have significant excess mortality from brain cancer. In 1995, brain cancer incidence was determined to increase among male farmers using pesticide in Sweden. These findings were confirmed by a population based case control study in eastern Nebraska. In this study, significant associations between some specific agricultural pesticide exposures and the risk of glioma among male farmers were demonstrated [128-134]. However, inconsistent studies are also available. A study from Norway determined no association between brain cancer incidence or mortality and agricultural pesticide usage. Population based case control studies from Sweden and United States found a non-significant increased risk of glioma with occupational pesticide use. One of the largest studies to date found no association between occupational pesticide exposure and glioma risk among men and women farmers. The relation between pesticide use and other types of cancer was also investigated. No significant associations were found between specific agricultural pesticide exposures and the risk of stomach or oesophageal adenocarcinomas among Nebraska farmers. [135-139]

Another professional group exposed to NOCs is clinical personels who handle alkylating chemotherapeutic agents and cancer patients treated with alkylating agent-based chemotherapy [7, 140, 141].

Drugs

Alkylating agents are one of the oldest anti-cancer drugs. They are still used in treatment of several types of cancer. The therapeutic drugs do not require metabolic activation. They cause both DNA alkylation and formation of cross-links between DNA strands. Alkylating drugs are generally methylating agents (e.g. temozolomide) or chloroethylating agents (e.g. carmustin and lomustine). Although O^6-methylguanine is major alkylation product, several other sites are also targets for alkylation. Firstly, chloroethylating agents form O^6-chloroethylguanine and other chloroethyl-adducts, and then at the O^6-position this is followed by dechlorination, formation of an unstable 1-O^6-ethanoguanine adduct and subsequent cross-linking between the ring nitrogens in 1-position of guanine and 3-position of cytosine (1-(3-cytosinyl)-2-(1-guanosinyl)-ethane).

Some alkylating drugs exert their strongest effects through alkylation of other positions and other types of cross-links. The effects of these drugs are strongly modulated by DNA repair processes [118, 119, 141, 142]. Categorization of alkylating anti-cancer drugs, their action mechanisms, resistance to these drugs and approaches to overcome the resistance is discussed in other chapters.

In addition to alkylating anti-cancer drugs, NOCs are formed by drugs containing various nitrosatable groups such as amines, amides and hydrazines which can react with nitrite in the acid medium of stomach. In an extensive study 182 drugs representing a wide variety of chemical structures were tested for their ability to react with nitrite, and 173 of them found to form NOCs and other reactive metabolites.

The problem of endogenous drug nitrosation is largely ignored. The exposure to drugs containing nitrosatable groups might be of greater attention than the exposure to NOCs containing foods. Because cured meats are the highest source of NOCs and they contain NOCs at concentrations which were found to change between 10-1000 µg/kg. The exposure to nitrosatable amines is below 100 mg/day with a normal diet. However certain nitrosatable drugs are used therapeutically at doses higher than 100 mg/day. Especially, paracetamol which is a secondary amine can reach the daily dose of 4 g [143, 144].

Conclusions

Animal and human studies investigating carcinogenic effect of NOCs were started in early 1960's. From that time to present much has been discovered. Many oncogenes and tumor suppressor genes were determined. Associations between genetic alterations in these genes and parallel impairments in biochemical networks were recognized. Role of epigenetic changes in carcinogenesis was discovered. In the light of improvements, carcinogenic mechanism of alkylating agents was revealed by animal studies in a certain manner. Epidemiological and case-control studies examining the association between NOCs and risk of brain, esophageal, stomach, nasopharynx, pancreas and colon cancers increased day to day. The evidence accumulated to date indicate carcinogenic impact of NOCs in humans. However, inconsistent findings are also available, this link was not supported by all studies. Probably, some investigations might be failed to provide information on levels of exposure. Some studies were based on a proxy exposure. All investigations based on estimated exposures by selected high NOCs containing food sources. The disadvantage of this approach was that much more frequently used foods with low to moderate N-nitroso content were not taken into consideration. In order to make an appropriate estimation of the total daily intake of NOCs for each individual summing values for that compounds from all food sources and from environment should be considered. Exposure concentrations of NOCs are known to vary by food source, food preparation and processing methods, planting area and growth conditions of consumed vegetables, nitrate content of drinking water and other environmental determinants such as work place and over time of individuals. Polymorphisms in N-nitroso compounds-metabolizing genes are also determinative for carcinogenicity of NOCs. Furthermore, it is important to determine to what extent nitrosation occurs in vivo, especially in the cases suffering from chronic inflammatory diseases. In this situation making an interpretation may be difficult. Significant associations determined by epidemiological and case-control studies may not evidence a cause-effect relationship.

However, on account of O^6-methylguanine adduct formed by NOCs has mutagenic potential and may play a role in cancer development, findings of the studies support the plausibility of a relation between NOCs exposure and cancer.

Diminishing human exposure to these carcinogens is one approach to prevention of cancer. Various medical and non-medical organisations were emphasized the carcinogenic potential of alkylating agent containing foods. Some precautions were taken to diminish the alkylating agent exposure so far. Looking ahead, there are various ways in which exposure of humans to NOCs can be decreased:

- Eating habits can be modificated
- Smoking and alcohol (especially beer) consumption can be stopped or tightly limited
- New technics which don't include alkylating agents can be investigated for food processing
- Hygienic and regulatory precautions can be currently imposed in occupational settings
- Daily consumption of various nitrosation inhibitors can be promoted
- Drinking water can be obtained from public water supplies instead of private wells
- Nitrosamine exposure can be monitored by sensitive methods in health centers
- Public awareness should be provided, especially in developing countries

Thus, lowering the body exposure to alkylating agents it is possible to reduce the risk of cancer a little bit.

Acknowledgments

The author thanks Onur Baykara for English review and Armagan Caglayan for her assistance in the organisation of references, figures and tables.

References

[1] IARC (2010) Agents Classified by the IARC Monographs, Volumes 1-1000. http://monographs .iarc.fr/ENG/Classification/Classifications GroupOrder.pdf

[2] Dietrich, M; Block, G; Pogoda, JM; Buffler, P; Hecht, S; Preston-Martin, S. A review: dietary and endogenously formed N-nitroso compounds and risk of childhood brain tumors. *Cancer Causes Control,* 2005 16(6), 619-635.

[3] Mirvish, SS. Role of N-nitroso compounds (NOC) and N-nitrosation in etiology of gastric, esophageal, nasopharyngeal and bladder cancer and contribution to cancer of known exposures to NOC. *Cancer Lett.,* 1995 93(1), 17-48.

[4] de Kok, TM; van Maanen, JM. Evaluation of fecal mutagenicity and colorectal cancer risk. *Mutat. Res.* 2000 463(1), 53-101.

[5] Magee, PN; Barnes, JM. The production of malignant primary hepatic tumours in the rat by feeding dimethylnitrosamine. *Br. J. Cancer,* 1956 10(1), 114-22.

[6] Umbenhauer, D; Wild, CP; Montesano, R; Saffhill, R; Boyle, JM; Huh, N; Kirstein, U; Thomale, J; Rajewsky, MF; Lu, SH. O(6)-methyldeoxyguanosine in oesophageal DNA among individuals at high risk of oesophageal cancer. *Int. J. Cancer,* 1985 36(6), 661-665.

[7] Reh, BD; DeBord, DG; Butler, MA; Reid, TM; Mueller, C; Fajen, JM. O(6)-methylguanine DNA adducts associated with occupational nitrosamine exposure. *Carcinogenesis,* 2000 21(1), 29-33.

[8] Janion, C. Inducible SOS response system of DNA repair and mutagenesis in Escherichia coli. *Int. J. Biol. Sci.,* 2008 4(6), 338-344.

[9] Franco, R; Schoneveld, O; Georgakilas, AG; Panayiotidis, MI. Oxidative stress, DNA methylation and carcinogenesis. *Cancer Lett.,* 2008 266(1), 6-11.

[10] Burns, JA; Dreij, K, Cartularo, L; Scicchitano, DA. O6-methylguanine induces altered proteins at the level of transcription in human cells. *Nucleic. Acids Res.,* 2010 38(22), 8178-8187.

[11] Pegg, AE. Multifaceted Roles of Alkyltransferase and Related Proteins in DNA Repair, DNA Damage, Resistance to Chemotherapy, and Research Tools. *Chem. Res. Toxicol.,* 2011 24(5), 618-639.

[12] Engelward, BP; Allan, JM; Dreslin, AJ; Kelly, JD; Wu, MM; Gold, B; Samson, LD. A chemical and genetic approach together define the

biological consequences of 3-methyladenine lesions in the mammalian genome. *J. Biol. Chem.*, 1998 273(9), 5412-5418.

[13]   Shrivastav, N; Li, D; Essigmann, JM. Chemical biology of mutagenesis and DNA repair: cellular responses to DNA alkylation. *Carcinogenesis*, 2010 31(1), 59-70.

[14]   Xu, Y; Sugiyama, H. Formation of the G-quadruplex and i-motif structures in retinoblastoma susceptibility genes (Rb). *Nucleic. Acids Res.*, 2006 34(3), 949-954.

[15]   Trewick, SC; Henshaw, TF; Hausinger, RP; Lindahl, T; Sedgwick, B. Oxidative demethylation by Escherichia coli AlkB directly reverts DNA base damage. *Nature*, 2002 419(6903), 174-178.

[16]   Falnes, PØ; Johansen, RF; Seeberg, E. AlkB-mediated oxidative demethylation reverses DNA damage in Escherichia coli. *Nature*, 2002 419(6903), 178-182.

[17]   Delaney, JC; Essigmann, JM. Mutagenesis, genotoxicity, and repair of 1-methyladenine,   3-alkylcytosines,   1-methylguanine,   and   3-methylthymine in alkB Escherichia coli. *Proc. Natl. Acad. Sci. USA*, 2004 101(39), 14051-14506.

[18]   Ishizaki, K; Tsujimura, T; Fujio, C; Zhang, YP; Yawata, H, Nakabeppu, Y, Sekiguchi, M, Ikenaga, M. Expression of the truncated E. coli O6-methylguanine methyltransferase gene in repair-deficient human cells and restoration of cellular resistance to alkylating agents. *Mutat. Res.*, 1987 184(2), 121-128.

[19]   Myers, LC; Jackow, F; Verdine, GL. Metal dependence of transcriptional switching in Escherichia coli Ada. *J. Biol. Chem.*, 1995 270(12), 6664-6670.

[20]   Pegg, AE. Repair of O6-alkylguanine by alkyltransferases. *Mutat. Res.*, 2000 462, 83–100.

[21]   Horiguchi, M; Kim, J; Matsunaga, N; Kaji, H; Egawa, T; Makino, K; Koyanagi, S; Ohdo, S. Glucocorticoid-dependent expression of O6-methylguanine-DNA methyltransferase genemodulates dacarbazine induced hepatotoxicity in mice. *J Pharmacol Exp Ther*, 2010 333, 782–787.

[22]   Dumenco, LL; Allay, E; Norton, K; Gerson, SL. The prevention of thymic lymphomas in transgenic mice by human O6-alkylguanine-DNA alkyltransferases. *Science*, 1993 259, 219–222.

[23]   Nakatsuru, Y; Matsukuma, S; Nemoto, N; Sugano, H; Sekiguchi, M; Ishikawa, T. O6-methylguanine-DNA methyltransferase protects against

nitrosamine-induced hepatocarcingenesis. *Proc. Natl. Acad. Sci*, 1993 90, 6468–6472.

[24] Becker, K; Gregel, CM; Kaina, B. The DNA repair protein O6-methylguanine-DNA methyltransferase protects against skin tumor formation induced by antineoplastic chloroethylnitrosourea. *Cancer Res.*, 1993 57, 3335–3338.

[25] Zaidi, NH; Pretlow, TP; O'Riordan, MA; Dumenco, LL; Allay, E; Gerson, SL. Transgenic expression of human MGMT protects against azoxymethane-induced aberrant crypt foci and G to A mutations in the K-ras oncogene of mouse colon. *Carcinogenesis*, 1995 16, 451–456.

[26] Liu, L; Qin, X; Gerson, SL. Reduced lung tumorigenesis in human methylguanine DNA-methyltransferase transgenic mice achieved by expression of transgene within the target cell. *Carcinogenesis*, 1999 20, 279–284.

[27] Iwakuma, T; Sakumi, K; Nakatsuru, Y; Kawate, H; Igarashi, H; Shiraishi, A; Tsuzuki, T; Ishikawa, T; Sekiguchi, M. High incidence of nitrosamine-induced tumorigenesis in mice lacking DNA repair methyltransferase. *Carcinogenesis*, 1997 18, 1631–1635.

[28] Bugni, JM; Meira, LB; Samson, LD. Alkylation induced colon tumorigenesis in mice deficient in the Mgmt and Msh6 proteins. *Oncogene*, 2008 28, 734–741.

[29] Nagasubramanian, R; Hansen, RJ; Delaney, SM; Cherian, MM; Samson, LD; Kogan, SC; Dolan, ME. Survival and tumorigenesis in O6-methylguanine DNA methyltransferase-deficient mice following cyclophosphamide exposure. *Mutagenesis*, 2008 23, 341–346.

[30] Klapacz, J; Meira, LB; Luchetti, DG; Calvo, JA; Bronson, RT; Edelmann, W; Samson, LD. O6-Methylguanine induced cell death involves exonuclease 1 as well as DNA mismatch recognition in vivo. *Proc. Natl. Acad. Sci USA*, 2009 106, 576–581.

[31] Gefen, N; Brkic, G; Galron, D; Priel, E; Ozer, J; Benharroch, D; Gopas, J. Acquired resistance to 6-thioguanine in melanoma cells involves the repair enzyme O6-methylguanine-DNA methyltransferase (MGMT). *Cancer Biol. Ther.*, 2010 9, 49–55.

[32] Waters, TR; Swann, PF. Cytotoxic mechanism of 6-thioguanine:hMutSa, the human mismatch binding heterodimer, binds to DNA containing S6-methylguanine. *Biochemistry*, 1997 36, 2501–2506.

[33] Spratt, TE; Campbell, CR. Synthesis of oligonucleotides containing analogs of O6-methylguanine and reaction with O6-alkylguanine-DNA alkyltransferase. *Biochemistry*, 1994 33, 11364–11371.

[34] Esteller, M; Toyota, M; Sanchez-Cespedes, M; Capella, G; Peinado, MA; Watkins, DN; Issa, JP; Sidransky, D; Baylin, SB; Herman, JG. Inactivation of the DNA repair gene O6-methylguanine-DNA methyltransferase by promoter hypermethylation is associated with G to A mutations in K-ras in colorectal tumorigenesis. *Cancer Res.*, 2000 60(9), 2368-2371.

[35] Esteller, M; Hamilton, SR; Burger, PC; Baylin, SB; Herman, JG. Inactivation of the DNA repair gene O6-methylguanine-DNA methyltransferase by promoter hypermethylation is a common event in primary human neoplasia. *Cancer Res.*, 1999 59, 793–797.

[36] Lai, JC; Cheng, YW; Goan, YG; Chang, JT; Wu, TC; Chen, CY; Lee, H. Promoter methylation of O6-methylguanine-DNA-methyltransferase in lung cancer is regulated by p53. *DNA Repair*, 2008 7, 1352–1363.

[37] Lai, JC; Wu, JY; Cheng, YW; Yeh, KT; Wu, TC; Chen, CY; Lee, H. O6-Methylguanine-DNA methyltransferase hypermethylation modulated by 17beta-estradiol in lung cancer cells. *Anticancer Res.*, 2009 29, 2535–2540.

[38] Bobustuc, GC; Baker, CH, Limaye, A; Jenkins, WD; Pearl, G; Avgeropoulos, NG; Konduri, SD. Levetiracetam enhances p53-mediated MGMT inhibition and sensitizes glioblastoma cells to Temozolomide. *Neuro-Oncology*, 2010 12, 917–927.

[39] Zhong, Y; Huang, Y; Zhang, T; Ma, C; Zhang, S; Fan, W; Chen, H; Qian, J; Lu, D. Effects of O6-methylguanine-DNA methyltransferase (MGMT) polymorphisms on cancer: a meta-analysis. *Mutagenesis*, 2010 25, 83–95.

[40] Liu, H; Xu-Welliver, M; Pegg, AE. The role of human O6-alkylguanine-DNA alkyltransferase in promoting 1,2-dibromoethane- induced genotoxicity in Escherichia coli. *Mutat. Res.*, 2010 452, 1–10.

[41] Liu, L; Pegg, AE; Williams, KM; Guengerich, FP. Paradoxical enhancement of the toxicity of 1,2-dibromoethane by O6- alkylguanine-DNA alkyltransferase. *J. Biol. Chem.*, 2002 277, 37920–37928.

[42] Liu, L; Hachey, DL; Valadez, G; Williams, KM; Guengerich, FP; Loktionova, NA; Kanugula, S; Pegg, AE. Characterization of a mutagenic DNA adduct formed from 1,2-dibromoethane by O6-alkylguanine-DNA alkyltransferase. *J. Biol. Chem.*, 2004 279, 4250–4259.

[43] Guengerich, FP. Principles of covalent binding of reactive metabolites and examples of activation of bis-electrophiles by conjugation. *Arch. Biochem. Biophys.*, 2005 433, 369–378.

[44] Liu, L; Xu-Welliver, M; Kanugula, S; Pegg, AE. Inactivation and degradation of O6-alkylguanine-DNA alkyltransferase after reaction with nitric oxide. *Cancer Res.*, 2002 62, 3037–3043.

[45] Wei, W; Li, B; Hanes, MA; Kakar, S; Chen, X; Liu, L. S-nitrosylation from GSNOR deficiency impairs DNA repair and promotes hepatocarcinogenesis. *Sci. Transl. Med.*, 2010 2(19), 19ra13.

[46] Kitahori, Y; Naito, H; Konishi, N; Ohnishi, T; Shirai, T; Hiasa Y. Frequent mutations of Ki-ras codon 12 in N-bis (2-hydroxypropyl)-nitrosamine-initiated thyroid, kidney and lung tumors in Wistar rats. *Cancer Lett.*, 1995 96(2), 155-161.

[47] Iwakuma, T; Sakumi, K, Nakatsuru, Y; Kawate, H, Igarashi, H; Shiraishi, A; Tsuzuki, T; Ishikawa, T; Sekiguchi, M. High incidence of nitrosamine-induced tumorigenesis in mice lacking DNA repair methyltransferase. *Carcinogenesis*, 1997 18(8), 1631-1635.

[48] Sukumar, S; Notario, V; Martin-Zanca, D; Barbacid, M. Induction of mammary carcinomas in rats by nitroso-methylurea involves malignant activation of H-ras-1 locus by single point mutations. *Nature*, 1983 306, 658–661.

[49] Bos, JL. Ras oncogenes in human cancer: a review. *Cancer Res.*, 1989 49, 4682–4689.

[50] Lozano, JC; Nakazawa, H; Cross, MP; Cabral, R; Yamasaki, H.GrA mutations in p53 and Ha-ras genes in esophageal papillomas induced by *N*-nitrosomethylbenzylamine in two strains of rats. *Mol. Carcinogen*, 1994 9, 33–39.

[51] Park, TJ; Han, SU; Cho, YK; Paik, WK; Kim, YB; Lim, IK. Methylation of O(6)-methylguanine-DNA methyltransferase gene is associated significantly with K-ras mutation, lymph node invasion, tumor staging, and disease free survival in patients with gastric carcinoma. *Cancer*, 2001 92(11), 2760-2768.

[52] Kohya, N; Kitajima, Y; Kitahara, K; Miyazaki, K. Mutation analysis of K-ras and beta-catenin genes related to O6-methylguanin-DNA methyltransferase and mismatch repair protein status in human gallbladder carcinoma. *Int. J. Mol. Med.* 2003 11(1), 65-69.

[53] Esteller, M; Risques, RA; Toyota, M; Capella, G; Moreno, V; Peinado, MA; Baylin, SB; Herman, JG. Promoter hypermethylation of the DNA repair gene O(6)-methylguanine-DNA methyltransferase is associated with the presence of G:C to A:T transition mutations in p53 in human colorectal tumorigenesis. *Cancer Res.* 2001 61(12), 4689-4692.

[54] Nakamura, M; Watanabe, T; Yonekawa, Y; Kleihues, P; Ohgaki, H. Promoter methylation of the DNA repair gene MGMT in astrocytomas is frequently associated with G:C --> A:T mutations of the TP53 tumor suppressor gene. *Carcinogenesis.* 2001 22(10), 1715-1719.

[55] Wolf, P; Hu, YC; Doffek, K; Sidransky, D; Ahrendt, SA. O(6)-Methylguanine-DNA methyltransferase promoter hypermethylation shifts the p53 mutational spectrum in non-small cell lung cancer. *Cancer Res.* 2001 61(22), 8113-8117.

[56] Yin, D; Xie, D; Hofmann, WK; Zhang, W; Asotra, K; Wong, R; Black, KL; Koeffler, HP. DNA repair gene O6-methylguanine-DNA methyltransferase: promoter hypermethylation associated with decreased expression and G:C to A:T mutations of p53 in brain tumors. *Mol Carcinog.* 2003 36(1), 23-31.

[57] Zhang, L; Lu, W; Miao, X; Xing, D; Tan, W; Lin, D. Inactivation of DNA repair gene O6-methylguanine-DNA methyltransferase by promoter hypermethylation and its relation to p53 mutations in esophageal squamous cell carcinoma. *Carcinogenesis.* 2003 24(6), 1039-1044.

[58] Maragos, CM; Hotchkiss, JH; Fubini, SL. Quantitative estimates of N-nitrosotrimethylurea formation in the porcine stomach. *Carcinogenesis.* 1990 11(9), 1587-1591.

[59] Mirvish, SS; Chu, C. Chemical determination of methylnitrosourea and ethylnitrosourea in stomach contents of rats, after intubation of the alkylureas plus sodium nitrite. *J. Natl. Cancer Inst.* 1973 50(3), 745-750.

[60] Sen, NP; Seaman, SW; Burgess, C; Baddoo, PA; Weber, D. Investigation on the possible formation of N-nitroso-N-methylurea by nitrosation of creatinine in model systems and in cured meats at gastric pH. *J. Agric. Food Chem.* 2000 48(10), 5088-5096.

[61] Sen, NP; Seaman, SW; Baddoo, PA; Burgess, C; Weber, D. Formation of N-nitroso-N-methylurea in various samples of smoked/dried fish, fish sauce, seafoods, and ethnic fermented/pickled vegetables following incubation with nitrite under acidic conditions. *J. Agric. Food Chem.* 2001 49(4), 2096-2103.

[62] Georgiadis, P; Samoli, E; Kaila, S; Katsouyanni, K; Kyrtopoulos, SA. Ubiquitous presence of O6-methylguanine in human peripheral and cord blood DNA. *Cancer Epidemiol. Biomarkers Prev.,* 2000 9(3), 299-305.

[63] Barrows, LR; Magee, PN. Nonenzymatic methylation of DNA by S-adenosylmethionine in vitro. *Carcinogenesis,* 1982 3, 349–351.

[64] Tricker, AR. N-nitroso compounds and man: sources of exposure, endogenous formation and occurrence in body fluids. *Eur. J. Cancer Prev.*, 1997 6(3), 226–268.

[65] Roediger, WW; Lawson, MJ; Radcliffe, BB. Nitrite from inflammatory cells - a cancer risk factor in ulcerative colitis. *Dis. Colon Rectum*, 1990 33, 1034–1036.

[66] Badawi, AF. Nitrate, nitrite and N-nitroso compounds in human bladder cancer associated with schistosomiasis. *Int. J. Cancer*, 2000 86(4), 598-600.

[67] Saad, AA; O'Connor, PJ; Mostafa, MH; Metwalli, NE; Cooper, DP; Margison, GP; Povey, AC. Bladder tumor contains higher N7-methylguanine levels in DNA than adjacent normal bladder epithelium. *Cancer Epidemiol. Biomarkers Prev.*, 2006 15(4), 740-743.

[68] Bartsch, H; Pignatelli, B; Calmels, S; Ohshima, H. Inhibition of nitrosation. *Basic Life Sci.*, 1993 61, 27-44.

[69] Vermeer, IT; Moonen, EJ; Dallinga, JW; Kleinjans, JC; van Maanen, JM. Effect of ascorbic acid and green tea on endogenous formation of N-nitrosodimethylamine and N-nitrosopiperidine in humans. *Mutat. Res.*, 1999 428(1-2), 353-361.

[70] Santarelli, RL; Pierre, F; Corpet, DE. Processed meat and colorectal cancer: a review of epidemiologic and experimental evidence. *Nutr. Cancer*, 2008 60(2), 131-144.

[71] Hughes, R; Cross, AJ; Pollock, JR; Bingham, S. Dose-dependent effect of dietary meat on endogenous colonic N-nitrosation. *Carcinogenesis*, 2001 22(1), 199-202.

[72] Bingham, SA; Hughes, R; Cross, AJ. Effect of white versus red meat on endogenous N-nitrosation in the human colon and further evidence of a dose response. *J. Nutr.*, 2002 132(11), 3522-3525.

[73] Cross, AJ; Pollock, JR; Bingham, SA. Haem, not protein or inorganic iron, is responsible for endogenous intestinal N-nitrosation arising from red meat. *Cancer Res.*, 2003 63(10), 2358-2360.

[74] Lunn, JC; Kuhnle, G; Mai, V; Frankenfeld, C; Shuker, DE; Glen, RC; Goodman, JM; Pollock, JR; Bingham, SA. The effect of haem in red and processed meat on the endogenous formation of N-nitroso compounds in the upper gastrointestinal tract. *Carcinogenesis*, 2007 28(3), 685-690.

[75] Bingham, S; Riboli, E. Diet and cancer-the European Prospective Investigation into Cancer and Nutrition. *Nat. Rev. Cancer*, 2004 4(3), 206-215.

[76] Sandhu, MS; White, IR; McPherson, K. Systematic review of the prospective cohort studies on meat consumption and colorectal cancer risk: a meta-analytical approach. *Cancer Epidemiol. Biomarkers Prev.*, 2001 10(5), 439-446.

[77] Norat, T; Lukanova, A; Ferrari, P; Riboli, E. Meat consumption and colorectal cancer risk: dose-response meta-analysis of epidemiological studies. *Int. J. Cancer*, 2002 98(2), 241-256.

[78] Larsson, SC; Wolk, A. Meat consumption and colorectal cancer risk: dose-response meta-analysis of epidemiological studies. *Int. J. Cancer*, 2006 119(11), 2657-2664.

[79] Chiu, BC; Gapstur, SM. Changes in diet during adult life and risk of colorectal adenomas. *Nutr. Cancer*, 2004 49(1), 49-58.

[80] Parnaud, G; Pignatelli, B; Peiffer, G; Taché, S; Corpet, DE. Endogenous N-nitroso compounds, and their precursors, present in bacon, do not initiate or promote aberrant crypt foci in the colon of rats. *Nutr. Cancer*, 2000 38(1), 74-80.

[81] Lijinsky, W. N-Nitroso compounds in the diet. *Mutat. Res.*, 1999 443(1-2), 129-138.

[82] Kuijten, RR; Bunin, GR; Nass, CC; Meadows, AT. Gestational and familial risk factors for childhood astrocytoma: results of a casecontrol study. *Cancer Res.*, 1990 50, 2608–2612.

[83] Bunin, GR; Kuitjen, RR; Buckley, JD; Rorke, LB; Meadows, AT. Relation between maternal diet and subsequent primitive neuroectodermal tumors in young children. *N. Engl. J. Med.*, 1993 329, 536–541.

[84] Baldwin, RT; Preston-Martin, S. Epidemiology of brain tumors in childhood-a review. Toxicol Appl Pharmacol, 2004 199(2), 118-131.

[85] Holick, CN; Giovannucci, EL; Rosner, B; Stampfer, MJ; Michaud, DS. Prospective study of intake of fruit, vegetables, and carotenoids and the risk of adult glioma. *Am. J. Clin. Nutr.*, 2007 85, 877–886.

[86] Terry, MB; Howe, G; Pogoda, JM; Zhang, FF; Ahlbom, A; Choi, W; Giles, GG; Little, J; Lubin, F; Menegoz, F; Ryan, P; Schlehofer, B; Preston-Martin, S. An international case-control study of adult diet and brain tumor risk: a histology-specific analysis by food group. *Ann. Epidemiol.*, 2009 19,161–171.

[87] Michaud, DS; Holick, CN; Batchelor, TT; Giovannucci, E; Hunter, DJ. Prospective study of meat intake and dietary nitrates, nitrites, and nitrosamines and risk of adult glioma. *Am. J. Clin. Nutr.*, 2009 90, 570–577.

[88] Dubrow, R; Darefsky, AS; Park, Y; Mayne, ST; Moore, SC; Kilfoy, B; Cross, AJ; Sinha, R; Hollenbeck, AR; Schatzkin, A; Ward, MH. Dietary components related to N-nitroso compound formation: a prospective study of adult glioma. *Cancer Epidemiol. Biomarkers Prev.*, 2010 19(7), 1709-1722.

[89] Hord, NG; Tang, Y; Bryan, NS. Food sources of nitrates and nitrites: the physiologic context for potential health benefits. *Am. J. Clin. Nutr.*, 2009 90(1), 1-10.

[90] World Cancer Research Fund. Food, nutrition, physical activity, and the prevention of cancer: a global perspective. Second Expert Report, 2007. Available from: http://www.dietandcancerreport.org

[91] Stuff, JE; Goh, ET; Barrera, SL; Bondy, ML; Forman, MR. Construction of an N-nitroso database for assessing dietary intake. *J. Food Compost Anal.*, 2009 22(1), 42-47.

[92] Chiu, BC; Ji, BT; Dai, Q; Gridley, G; McLaughlin, JK; Gao, YT; Fraumeni, JF Jr; Chow, WH. Dietary factors and risk of col. on cancer in Shanghai, China. *Cancer Epidemiol. Biomarkers Prev.*, 2003 12(3), 201-208.

[93] Ward, MH. Too much of a good thing? Nitrate from nitrogen fertilizers and cancer. *Rev. Environ. Health*, 2009 24(4), 357-363.

[94] De Roos, AJ; Ward, MH; Lynch, CF; Cantor, KP. Nitrate in public water supplies and the risk of colon and rectum cancers. *Epidemiology*, 2003 14(6), 640-649.

[95] World Health Organization. Recommendations; nitrate and nitrite. In:Guidelines for drinking water quality. 3rd ed Geneva, Switzerland:WHO, 2004.

[96] United States Environmental Protection Agency. 2003. Available from: http:// www.epa.gov/ safewater/ sdwa/ sdwa.html.

[97] Moller, H; Landt, J; Pedersen, E; Jensen, P; Autrup, H; Jensen, OM. Endogenous nitrosation in relation to nitrate exposure from drinking water and diet in a Danish rural population. *Cancer Res.*, 1989 49, 3117–3121.

[98] Mirvish, SS; Grandjean, AC; Moller, H; Fike, S; Maynard, T; Jones, L; Rosinsky, S; Nie, G. N-nitrosoproline excretion by rural Nebraskans drinking water of varied nitrate content. *Cancer Epidemiol. Biomarkers Prev.*, 1992 1, 455–461.

[99] Rowland, IR; Granli, T; Bockman, OC; Key, PE; Massey, RC. Endogenous N-nitrosation inman assessed by measurement of apparent

total N-nitroso compounds in faeces. *Carcinogenesis,* 1991 12, 1395–1401.

[100] Vermeer, ITM; Pachen, DMFA; Dallinga, JW; Kleinjans, JCS; van Maanen, JMS. Volatile *N*-nitrosamine formation after intake of nitrate at the ADI level in combination with an amine-rich diet, *Environ. Health Perspect,* 1998 106, 459–463.

[101] Cuello, C; Correa, P; Haenszel, W; Gordillo, G; Brown, C; Archer, M; Tannenbaum, S. Gastric cancer in Colombia: I. Cancer risk and suspect environmental agents, *J. Natl. Cancer Inst.,* 1976 56, 1015–1020.

[102] Gilli, G; Corrao, G; Favilli, S. Concentrations of nitrates in drinking water and incidence of gastric carcinomas: first descriptive study of the Piemonte region, Italy, *Sci. Total Environ,* 1984 34, 35–48.

[103] Morales Suarez-Varela, MM; Llopis-Gonzalez, A; Tejerizo-Perez, ML. Impact of nitrates in drinking water on cancer mortality in Valencia, Spain. *Eur. J. Epidemiol.,* 1995 11, 15–21.

[104] Van Leeuwen, JA; Waltner-Toews, D; Abernathy, T; Smit, B; Shoukri, M. Associations between stomach cancer and drinking water contamination with atrazine and nitrate in Ontario (Canada) agroecosystems, 1987–1991. *Int. J. Epidemiol.,* 1999 28, 836–840.

[105] Gulis, G; Czompolyova, M; Cerhan, JR. An ecologic study of nitrate in municipal drinking water and cancer incidence in Trnava district, Slovakia. *Environ Res.,* 2002 88, 182–187.

[106] Volkmer, BG; Ernst, B; Simon, J; Kuefer, R; Bartsch, G Jr; Bach, D; Gschwend, JE. Influence of nitrate levels in drinking water on urological malignancies: a community-based cohort study. *BJU Int.,* 2005 95, 972–976.

[107] Weyer, PJ; Cerhan, JR; Kross, BC; Hallberg, GR; Kantamneni, J; Breuer, G; Jones, MP; Zheng, W; Lynch, CF. Municipal drinking water nitrate level and cancer risk in older women: the Iowa Women's Health Study. *Epidemiology,* 2001 12, 327–338.

[108] Boeing, H; Frentzel-Beyme, F. Regional risk factors for stomach cancer in the FRG. *Environ. Health Perspect,* 1991 94, 83–89.

[109] Kross, BC; Hallberg, GR; Bruner, DR; Cherryholmes, K; Johnson, JK. The nitrate contamination of private well water in Iowa. *Am. J. Public Health,* 1993 83, 270–272.

[110] Ward, MH; Cantor, KP; Riley, D; Merkle, S; Lynch, CF. Nitrate in public water supplies and risk of bladder cancer. *Epidemiology,* 2003 14(2), 183-190.

[111] Lijinsky, W. N-Nitroso compounds in the diet. *Mutation Research*, 1999 443, 129–138.

[112] Andersopn, LM; Koseniauskas, R; Burak, ES; Logsdon, DL; Carter, JP; Driver, CL; Gombar, CT; Magee, PN; Harrington, GW. Suppression of in vivo clearance of N-nitrosodimethylamine in mice with cotreatment with ethanol. *Drug Metab. Dispos*, 1994 22, 43-49.

[113] Anderson, LM; Souliotis, VL; Chhabra, SK; Moskal, TJ; Harbaugh, SD, Kyrtopoulos, SA. N-nitrosodimethylamine-derived O(6)-methylguanine in DNA of monkey gastrointestinal and urogenital organs and enhancement by ethanol. *Int. J. Cancer*, 1996 66, 130-134.

[114] Espina, N; Lima, V; Lieber, CS; Garro, AJ. In vitro and in vivo inhibitory effect of ethanol and acetaldehyde on O6- methylguanine transferase. *Carcionogenesis*, 1988 9, 761–766.

[115] Pöschl, G; Seitz, HK. Alcohol and cancer. *Alcohol Alcohol*, 2004 39(3), 155-165.

[116] Grosse, Y; Baan, R; Straif, K, Secretan, B; El Ghissassi, F; Cogliano, V. Carcinogenicity of nitrate, nitrite, and cyanobacterial peptide toxins. *Lancet Oncol*, 2006 7(8), 628–629.

[117] Lijinsky, W. The significance of N-nitroso compounds as environmental carcinogens. *J. Environ. Sci. Health*, 1986 C4(1), 1–45.

[118] Barsch, H; Montesano, R. Relevance of nitrosamines to human cancer. *Carcinogenesis*, 1984 5(11), 1381-1383.

[119] 19. Drabløs, F; Feyzi, E; Aas, PA; Vaagbø, CB; Kavli, B; Bratlie, MS; Peña-Diaz, J; Otterlei, M; Slupphaug, G; Krokan, HE. Alkylation damage in DNA and RNA--repair mechanisms and medical significance. *DNA Repair* (Amst), 2004 3(11), 1389-1407.

[120] Hecht, SS. Cigarette smoking and lung cancer: chemical mechanisms and approaches to prevention. *Lancet Oncol.*, 2002 3(8), 461–469.

[121] Akopyan, G; Bonavida, B. Understanding tobacco smoke carcinogen NNK and lung tumorigenesis. *Int. J. Oncol.*, 2006 29(4), 745–752.

[122] Pulling, LC; Klinge, DM; Belinsky, SA. p16INK4a and beta-catenin alterations in rat liver tumors induced by NNK. *Carcinogenesis*, 2001 22(3), 461–466.

[123] Vuillemenot, BR; Hutt, JA; Belinsky, SA. Gene promoter hypermethylation in mouse lung tumors. *Mol. Cancer Res.*, 2006 4(4), 267–273.

[124] Lin, RK; Hsieh, YS; Lin, P; Hsu, HS; Chen, CY; Tang, YA; Lee, CF; Wang, YC. The tobacco-specific carcinogen NNK induces DNA methyltransferase 1 accumulation and tumor suppressor gene

hypermethylation in mice and lung cancer patients. *J. Clin. Invest.*, 2010 120(2), 521-532.

[125] Carmella, SG; Borukhova, A; Desai, D; Hecht, SS; Evidence for endogenous formation of tobacco-specific nitrosamines in rats treated with tobacco alkaloids and sodium nitrite. *Carcinogenesis*, 1997 18, 587–592.

[126] Tyroller, S; Zwickenpflug, W; Richter, E. New sources of dietary myosmine uptake from cereals, fruits, vegetables, and milk. *J. Agric. Food Chem.*, 2002 50, 4909–4915.

[127] Raj, A; Mayberry, JF; Podas, T. Occupation and gastric cancer. *Postgrad Med. J.*, 2003 79(931), 252-258.

[128] Tricker, AR; Spiegelhalder, B; Preussman, R. Environmental exposure to preformed nitroso compounds. *Cancer Surveys*, 1989 8, 251–272.

[129] Musicco, M; Sant, M; Molinari, S; Filippini, G; Gatta, G; Berrino, F. A case-control study of brain gliomas and occupational exposure to chemical carcinogens: the risk to farmers. *Am. J. Epidemiol.*, 1988 128, 778–785.

[130] Koestner, A. Characterization of N-nitrosourea-induced tumors of the nervous system; their prospective value for studies of neurocarcinogenesis and brain tumor therapy. *Toxicol. Pathol.*, 1990 18, 186–192.

[131] Figa-Talamanca, I; Mearelli, I; Valente, P; Bascherini, S. Cancer mortality in a cohort of rural licensed pesticide users in the province of Rome. *Int. J. Epidemiol.*, 1993 22, 579–583.

[132] Kross, BC; Burmeister, LF; Ogilvie, LK; Fuortes, LJ; Fu, CM. Proportionate mortality study of golf course superintendents. *Am. J. Ind. Med.*, 1996 29, 501–506.

[133] Wiklund, K; Dich, J. Cancer risks among male farmers in Sweden. *Eur. J. Cancer Prev.*, 1995 4, 81–90.

[134] Lee, WJ; Colt, JS; Heineman, EF; McComb, R; Weisenburger, DD; Lijinsky, W; Ward, MH. Agricultural pesticide use and risk of glioma in Nebraska, United States. *Occup. Environ. Med.*, 2005 62(11), 786-792.

[135] Kristensen, P; Andersen, A; Irgens, LM; Laake, P; Bye, AS. Incidence and risk factors of cancer among men and women in Norwegian agriculture. *Scand. J. Work Environ Health*, 1996 22, 14–26.

[136] Rodvall, Y; Ahlbom, A; Spannare, B, Nise, G. Glioma and occupational exposure in Sweden, a case-control study. *Occup Environ Med*, 1996 53, 526–537.

[137] De Roos, AJ; Stewart, PA; Linet, MS; Heineman, EF; Dosemeci, M; Wilcosky, T; Shapiro, WR; Selker, RG; Fine, HA; Black, PM; Inskip, PD. Occupation and the risk of adult glioma in the United States. *Cancer Causes Control*, 2003 14, 139–150.

[138] Schlehofer, B; Hettinger, I; Ryan, P; Blettner, M; Preston-Martin, S; Little, J; Arslan, A; Ahlbom, A; Giles, GG; Howe, GR; Ménégoz, F; Rodvall, Y; Choi, WN; Wahrendorf, J. Occupational risk factors for low grade and high grade glioma: results from an international case control study of adult brain tumours. *Int. J. Cancer*, 2005 113, 116–125.

[139] Lee, WJ; Lijinsky, W; Heineman, EF; Markin, RS; Weisenburger, DD; Ward, MH. Agricultural pesticide use and adenocarcinomas of the stomach and oesophagus. *Occup. Environ. Med.*, 2004 61(9), 743-749.

[140] Oesch, F; Klein, S. Relevance of environmental alkylating agents to repair protein O6-alkylguanine-DNA alkyltransferase: determination of individual and collective repair capacities of O6-methylguanine. *Cancer Res.*, 1992 52(7), 1801-1803.

[141] Leone, G; Fianchi, L; Pagano, L; Voso, MT. Incidence and susceptibility to therapy-related myeloid neoplasms. *Chem. Biol. Interact*, 2010 184(1-2), 39-45.

[142] Margison, GP; Santibañez-Koref, MF; Povey, AC. Mechanisms of carcinogenicity/ chemotherapy by O6-methylguanine. *Mutagenesis,* 2002 17, 483–487.

[143] Nielsen, JB; Lings, S. Nitrosamine formation via non-prescription drugs? *Med. Hypotheses*, 1994 42(4), 265-278.

[144] Brambilla, G; Martelli, A. Genotoxic and carcinogenic risk to humans of drug-nitrite interaction products. *Mutat. Res.*, 2007 635(1), 17-52.

In: Alkylating Agents …
Editor: Yildiz Dincer

ISBN: 978-1-62618-487-9
© 2013 Nova Science Publishers, Inc.

Chapter III

Alkylating Agents
in Chemotherapy

Tiraje Celkan[*]

Istanbul University Cerrahpasa Medical Faculty,
Department of Pediatric Hematology, Istanbul, Turkey

Abstract

Alkylating agents are the oldest class of anticancer agents. They were known for their use as "mustard gas" for chemical weapons in World War I. Although each day a new targeted therapy is found, they are still the backbone of regimens of newly diagnosed or refractory diseases of every kind of cancer in both adults and children. Alkylating agents are a class of chemotherapy drugs that bind to DNA and prevent proper DNA replication. They have chemical groups that can form permanent covalent bonds with nucleophilic sites in the DNA. Alkylating agents involve reactions mainly with guanine in DNA. They add alkyl groups to DNA bases which results fragmentation due to repair activity. A second mechanism is the formation of cross-bridges in the DNA which could not be separated for synthesis or transcription. The third mechanism is the mispairing of the nucleotides leading to mutations. There are six groups of alkylating agents: nitrogen mustards; ethylenimes; alkylsulfonates; triazenes; piperazines; and nitrosureas. Usually tumors that are resistant to conventional agents are disappeared by a complex mechanism of

[*] E-mail: tirajecelkan@yahoo.com.

action of alkylating agents, so they are one of the major alternatives for the clinicians.

In this chapter, we review the major classes of alkylating agents used in chemotherapy regimens, mainly their mechanism of action and members of new generations.

Introduction

Depending on their characteristics and effects, chemotherapy agents can be categorized as alkylating agents, antimetabolites, anthracyclines, antitumor antibiotics, monoclonal antibodies, platinums, or plant alkaloids. Most chemotherapy agents and medications are effective by interfering with DNA synthesis or function. Based on their chemical action at a cellular phase, chemotherapy agents can be classified as cell-cycle specific agents or cell-cycle nonspecific agents. Alkylating drugs are non-hormonal chemotherapeutics which are effective during all phases of cell cycle. Therefore, they are used to treat a large number of cancers. However, they are usually more successful in treating slow-growing cancers, especially in solid tumors and leukemia [1-4]. The alkyl group is attached to the guanine base of DNA, at number 7 nitrogen atom of the purine ring [1]. Hyperthermia is especially effective at enhancing the effects of alkylating agents [2]. Usually cancer cells proliferate faster with more error. Because their error-correction mechanism is not as perfect as healthy cells. This situation makes cancer cells more sensitive to DNA damage (being alkylated). Alkylating agents are toxic to normal cells leading to damage, especially in cells that divide frequently (gastrointestinal tract, bone marrow, testicles and ovaries). Long term use of alkylating agents can lead to permanent infertility by decreasing sperm production in males, and causing menstruation cessation in females. Alkylating agents are also carcinogenic. Many alkylating agents can also lead to secondary cancers such as acute myeloid leukemia, years after the therapy [4]. Before their use in chemotherapy, alkylating agents were better known for mustard gas which is related to chemical weapons in World War I [4]. The compound was used as a weapon because of its vesicant effects, which produce blindness, skin irritation and pulmonary damage. However, it was observed that people who were exposed to sulfur mustard also developed bone marrow suppression and lymphoid aplasia (After the accident in Bari, Italy, at 1943) [5-7]. Because of these findings, sulfur mustard was evaluated as the first cancer treatment agent [1]. Trials in patients with lymphoma demonstrated regression of tumors, with relief of symptoms [5]. The first use of alkylating agents for Hodgkin's disease lymphosarcoma, leukemia, and other malignancies resulted in striking but temporary involution of tumor masses. This result was not spoken till the end of World War II because of the secrecy, and was published in 1946 [5-7].

Action Mechanisms of Alkylating Agents

Alkylating agents involve reactions with guanine in DNA. These drugs add methyl or other alkyl groups onto molecules and cause miscoding of DNA [4]. In the *first* mechanism, an alkylating agent attaches alkyl groups to DNA bases. This alteration results in DNA fragmentation by repair enzymes in their attempts to remove the alkylated bases. A *second* mechanism of alkylating agents to cause DNA damage is the formation of cross-bridges between atoms in the DNA. In this process, two bases are linked together by an alkylating agent that has two DNA binding sites. Cross-linking prevents separation of DNA strands for replication or transcription. The *third* mechanism of action is mispairing of alkylated nucleotides leading to mutations.

Alkylating agents stop tumor growth by crosslinking guanine nucleobases in DNA double-helix strands. This makes the strands unable to uncoil and separate which are essential in DNA replication. Therefore cells can no longer divide. These drugs act nonspecifically *during all phases of cell cycle.* Monoalkylating agents can react only with one 7-N of guanine [2-4]. Dialkylating agents can react with two different 7-N-guanine residues, and, if this occurs on different strands of DNA, the result is cross-linkage of the DNA strands, which prevents uncoiling of the DNA double helix. If the two guanine residues are in the same strand, the result is called *limpet attachment* of the drug molecule to the DNA. Limpet attachment and monoalkylation do not prevent the separation of the two DNA strands of the double helix but prevent the access of vital DNA-processing enzymes into DNA molecule. The final result is inhibition of cell growth or stimulation of apoptosis, cell suicide.

Chemistry of the Alkylating Agents

The alkylating agents are the compounds that react with electron-rich atoms to form covalent bonds. They are divided into two types:

1.   those that react directly with biologic molecules (SN1)
2.   those that form an intermediate reactive, which then reacts with the
     biologic molecules (SN2) [4].

SN1 and SN2 type kinetics of the reactions are different as the rate of
reaction of an SN1 agent is dependent only on the concentration of the reactive
intermediate, whereas the rate of reaction of an SN2 agent is dependent on the
concentration of the alkylating agent and of the molecule reacting with DNA.
The nitrogen mustards and nitrosoureas are examples of SN1 agents, busulfan
is an SN2 agent.

Types of Alkylating Agents

Many of the agents are known as "*Classical alkylating agents*". These
include true alkyl groups. Classical alkylating agents are shown in the Table 1.

Platinum-based chemotherapeutic drugs act in a similar manner. These
agents do not have an alkyl group, but nevertheless damage DNA [4]. They
permanently coordinate to DNA to interfere with DNA repair, so they are
either described as "*alkylating-like*" or as nonclassical alkylating agents [4].

Platinum group includes (cisplatin, carboplatin, nedaplatin, oxaplatin,
satraplatin, triplatin tetranitrate). These agents also bind at N7 of guanine.
Certain alkylating agents are sometimes described as "nonclassical". They
include procarbazine, altretamine, tetrazines (dacarbazine, mitozolomide,
temozolomide) [4].

Table 1. Classical alkylating agents

Mechlorethamine or mustine (HN_2) Melphalan Chlorambucil Ifosfamide Nitrosoureas Carmustine Lomustine	Nitrogen mustards Cyclophosphamide Streptozotocin Alkyl sulfonates Busulfan Thiotepa *

* Thiotepa and its analogues are also considered as nonclassical alkylating agent by
  certain books.

Nitrogen Mustards

The most frequently used alkylating agents are the nitrogen mustards. Only five nitrogen mustards are commonly used in cancer therapy today. These are mechlorethamine, cyclophosphamide, ifosfamide, melphalan, and chlorambucil. All of the nitrogen mustards react through an aziridinium intermediate. Cyclophosphamide is one of the most potent immunosuppressive substances. In small dosages, it is also efficient in the therapy of autoimmune diseases. High dosages cause pancytopenia and hemorrhagic cystitis.

Alkylation Mechanism of Nitrogen Mustards

Cyclophosphamide is not a reactive compound, but it undergoes activation in the body. The initial activation reaction is carried out by cytochrome P450 mediated microsomal oxidation in the liver. The new compound 4-hydroxycyclophosphamide diffuses from the hepatocyte into the plasma and is distributed throughout the body. As 4-hydroxycyclophosphamide is a nonpolar metabolite, it enters target cells by diffusion. Aldophosphamide spontaneously decomposes to produce phosphoramide mustard, which is the first reactive alkylating agent produced in the metabolism of cyclophosphamide. Although phosphoramide mustard is also produced extracellularly, this compound is very polar, and enters cells poorly, and probably plays a minor role. Free chloroethylaziridine (cyclized form of phosphoramide mustard) may contribute significantly to the alkylation and cross-linking of DNA [2-4].

The toxic compound acrolein is produced by the metabolism of cyclophosphamide [8]. After administration of high doses of cyclophosphamide, a decrease in the enzyme O^6-alkyguanine-alkyltransferase in circulating lymphocytes has been detected [9]. The tumor cells with elevated O^6-alkylguanine-alkyltransferase have been sensitized to 4-hydroperoxycyclophosphamide by depletion of the enzyme [10]. Acrolein released by cyclophosphamide forms an O^6-guanyl adduct that can be removed by O^6-alkyguanine-alkyltransferase. Thus, acrolein contributes to the antitumor activity and probably the carcinogenic effects of cyclophosphamide, and these effects are abrogated by the action of O^6-alkylguanine-alkyltransferase.

Cyclophosphamide produces less gastrointestinal and hematopoietic toxicity than other alkylating agents do. The basis for this decreased toxicity is the enzyme aldehyde dehydrogenase [11]. This enzyme oxidizes aldophosphamide to carboxyphosphamide, an inactive product, which is excreted in the urine and accounts for about 80% of an administered dose of cyclophosphamide in any species. This enzyme is found in high concentration in the hepatic cytosol, primitive hematopoietic cells, stem cells and mucosal absorptive cells in the intestine. Administration of an inhibitor of this enzyme to an animal markedly increases the hematopoietic and gastrointestinal toxicity of cyclophosphamide.

Ifosfamide, a structural isomer of cyclophosphamide, is used particularly in the treatment of testicular tumors and sarcomas [12-14]. Ifosfamide undergoes the same metabolic reactions like as cyclophosphamide, but the location of the chloroethyl group on the ring nitrogen produces quantitative changes in the metabolism of the drug [15]. The primary metabolite, aldoifosfamide, is a substrate for aldehyde dehydrogenase. The side effects of this compound in bone marrow and gastrointestinal tract are similar to those of cyclophosphamide. The oxidation of the chloroethyl side chains to produce choroacetaldehyde is a minor metabolic pathway for cyclophosphamide (<10% of dose) but is increased to as much as 50% for ifosfamide [16]. Neurotoxicity of ifosfamide is the result of increased production of chloracetaldehyde [17] which may also contribute to the greater renal and bladder toxicity. Ifosfamide mustard has higher side chain oxidation and lesser reactivity, so clinically, ifosfamide is used at higher doses than cyclophosphamide.

Melphalan is an alkylating agent that is used extensively in the treatment of multiple myeloma [18], ovarian cancer [19] and breast cancer [20]. Melphalan is an amino acid analogue that has been shown to enter cells and cross the blood-brain barrier through active transport systems.

Chlorambucil is used extensively for the treatment of chronic lymphocytic leukemia [21], ovarian carcinoma, [22] and lymphoma [23] but it is used less often in high-dose combination therapies than the other nitrogen mustards that are described here. This agent is well tolerated and can be used in patients who have severe nausea and vomiting with other alkylating agents.

Aziridines and Epoxides

The aziridines (thiotepa, mitomycin C, and diaziquone) are the compounds which are closely related to nitrogen mustards. These agents presumably alkylate the DNA with the same mechanism as the aziridinium intermediates produced by the nitrogen mustards, but the aziridine rings in these compounds are uncharged and less reactive than aziridinium compounds.

Thiotepa (triethylene thiophosphoramide) is used in the treatment of carcinomas of the ovary and breast and for the intrathecal therapy of meningeal carcinomatosis [24]. Thiotepa is oxidatively desulfurated by hepatic microsomes to produce triethylene phosphoramide (TEPA) [25]. Although TEPA is less cytotoxic than thiotepa [26], after the clinical administration of thiotepa, both thiotepa and TEPA are present in the blood and the concentration and area under the curve (AUC) for TEPA exposure may exceed those of thiotepa [26]. The AUC exposure to thiotepa is correlated with the degree of myelo suppression in patients. It is thought that the activity of thiotepa is enhanced by low pH within tumor cells.

Mitomycin C is a natural product that is used in the treatment of breast cancer and cancers of the gastrointestinal tract [27, 28]. This compound contains an aziridine ring and effective through the cross-linking of DNA [4]. Following this alkylation, a displacement of the activated carbamate group on the number 10 carbon atom of mitomycin C by an extracyclic amino nitrogen of a guanylic acid molecule on the complementary DNA strand occurs to produce an interstrand DNA cross-link.

Diaziquone (AZQ) has been designed to be sufficiently lipophilic to readily cross the blood-brain barrier for the treatment of central nervous system (CNS) tumors [29]. It demonstrates clinical activity against brain tumors, other solid tumors, and leukemia. AZQ undergoes reduction of the quinone ring in cells. This reduction results in protonation of the aziridine rings and enhancement of reactivity of the compound.

The *epoxides* such as dianhydrogalactitol are chemically related to the aziridines and alkylate through a similar mechanism [30]. Dibromodulcitol is hydrolyzed to dianhydrogalactitol and thus is a pro-drug as an epoxide [31].

Alkyl Sulfonates

The alkyl alkane sulfonate busulfan is one of the earliest alkylating agents that alkylate through an SN2 reaction. In preclinical studies, hepsulfam, an alkyl sulfamate analogue of busulfan with a wider range of antitumor activity was evaluated in clinical trials [32] but was demonstrated no superiority to busulfan. Busulfan is the most interesting but poorly understood alkylating agent with its selective toxicity for early myeloid precursors [4]. This selective effect is probably responsible for its activity against chronic myelocytic leukemia (CML). The use of busulfan as first-line therapy for the treatment of CML was succeeded by the use of the less toxic hydroxyurea and, a targeted therapeutics with imatinib mesylate in last decade [33]. The current major use of busulfan is as a component of bone marrow ablative regimens for bone marrow and stem cell transplantation of patients with acute myeloid leukemia and other malignancies [34].

Nitrosoureas

The nitrosoureas are a class of alkylating agents which received considerable attention during the past three decades [4]. These compounds decompose to produce alkylating compounds under physiologic conditions. The agent is decomposed to chloroethyl diazonium, which was shown to react with DNA.

Carmustine (BCNU) was the first agent to demonstrate significant activity against a preclinical model of intracerebral tumor [35] and is currently used in the treatment of primary brain tumors and multiple myeloma. *Lomustine (CCNU)* and *Semustine (methyl CCNU)* demonstrated greater activity against solid tumors in preclinical studies. CCNU is used in the treatment of CNS tumors and lymphomas, and methyl CCNU is used particularly in the treatment of gastrointestinal tumors [2-4]. *ACNU*, which is more water soluble than most of the other nitrosoureas, is employed for the intra-arterial and intrathecal treatment of CNS tumors and the treatment of solid tumors. The clinical use of the nitrosoureas is limited by marked and *prolonged hematopoietic toxicity* and by renal toxicity [2].

Triazenes, Hydrazines

These are nitrogen-containing compounds that spontaneously decompose or can be metabolized to produce alkyl diazonium intermediates that alkylate biologic molecules. Procarbazine and dacarbazine, are metabolized to reactive intermediates that decompose to produce methyl diazonium, which methylates DNA.

It is most likely that the mechanism involving in the DNA methylation and subsequent cytotoxicity is the generation of methylazoxyprocarbazine. The activation of dacarbazine occurs via N-methyl oxidation by a microsomal P450 enzyme. Both procarbazine and dacarbazine are used in the treatment of Hodgkins disease [36].

Procarbazine is a component of combination regimens used for the treatment of primary brain tumors [37] and dacarbazine is used in the treatment of melanoma [38]. Procarbazine was originally developed as a monoamine oxidase inhibitor, and it can lead CNS depression and acute hypertensive reactions after the ingestion of tyramine-rich foods [39].

Temozolomide spontaneously decomposes under physiologic conditions to produce the same active metabolite produced by DTIC. Temozolomide, which is administered orally, has demonstrated antitumor activity against gliomas and melanomas [40].

Hexamethylmelamine is an active antitumor agent that is considered to be acting as an alkylating agent, because the methyl groups are required for antitumor activity. The methyl groups are hydroxylated with subsequent demethylation in vivo [41]. The agent is also significant antitumor activity against ovarian cancer.

Toxicities of Alkylating Agents

The characteristic toxicities of the alkylating agents are hematopoietic, gastrointestinal, gonadal, and CNS toxicity. However, each of the agents has a characteristic set of toxicities, determined by the reactivity, metabolism, and distribution of the agent, and the clinician should be aware of these idiosyncrasies of the agents.

Although the alkylating agents react with a number of biologic molecules, (amino acids, thiols, RNA, and DNA), the cytotoxic effects of the agents are due to reactions with DNA. Bifunctional agents are much more effective antitumor agents than monofunctional agents, but addition of more than two alkylating groups does not lead a further increase in cytotoxic activity. A good correlation was shown between cytotoxicity and the formation of interstrand cross-links by bifunctional alkylating agents. Although the alkylating agents can react with virtually all of the nitrogens in the DNA bases, there is a selectivity based on the electron density of the nitrogens and the local structure of the DNA. The nitrogen mustards react most readily with the N-7 position of guanylic acid. The reactive species of the nitrosoureas is more reactive than the aziridiniums of the nitrogen mustards and initially alkylates the 0-6 position of guanylic acid [4, 42].

Alkylating agents such as methylnitrosourea, procarbazine, and dacarbazine are not bifunctional and cause methylation of DNA, predominantly on the O-6 and N-7 positions of guanylic acid. These lesions can produce both spontaneous and enzyme-mediated single strand breaks, which are cytotoxic [2, 4].

Toxicity of Each Drug

Cyclophosphamide-Ifosfamide- The rate of the metabolism of this compound varies considerably among individuals and can be modulated by the administration compounds such as phenobarbital or a previous dose of cyclophosphamide that induce the rate of microsomal metabolism. However, usually it has a half-life of 3 to 10 hours at conventional doses and the clearance rate of the compound does not appear to be significantly affecting the toxicity or therapeutic effect of the agent [4, 42]. At higher doses currently being used in bone marrow transplantation regimens, however, the plasma concentrations of cyclophosphamide should be close to the capacity of the microsomal activating enzymes. Cyclophosphamide and ifosfamide can induce their own metabolism.

The majority of a dose of cyclophosphamide (< 70%) is excreted in the urine as the inactive metabolite carboxyphosphamide [43]. Renal function does not significantly affect the toxicity of cyclophosphamide [44] most likely because of spontaneous decomposition, and absence of renal excretion. The clinical pharmacology of ifosfamide is similar to that of cyclophosphamide. As compared to same dose of cyclophosphamide, lower systemic concentrations of the 4-hydroxy metabolite are achieved for ifosfamide [45]. Both cyclophosphamide and ifosfamide are well absorbed after oral administration [46].

Melphalan- Plasma peak level of 4 to 13 micromolar is present after intravenous administration of a 0.6 mg/kg dose of melphalan, and the half-life (t1/2b) is 1.8 hours [47]. There is variable systemic availability after oral dosing [48], and it was shown that oral administration of foods with melphalan inhibits absorption of the agent. It was reported that myelosuppression by melphalan is increased in patients with decreased renal function.

Chlorambucil- After the oral administration of 0.6 mg/kg of chlorambucil, plasma peak level of 2 to 6 micromolar at the first hour for parent compound, and peak level of 2 to 4 micromolar at 2 to 4 hours after chlorambucil administration for phenylacetic acid mustard are determined. The plasma half-life of chlorambucil is 92 minutes and that of phenylacetic acid mustard is 145 minutes.

Thiotepa- After an intravenous injection of 12 mg/m^2 thiotepa, plasma peak level of about 5 micromolar is achieved and thiotepa is found to decay with a plasma half-life of 125 minutes. TEPA remains in plasma longer than thiotepa. When given intraperitoneally, the concomitant increase in plasma level is associated to the same dose obtained by intravenous administration

[49]. After intravenous injection, comparable cerebrospinal fluid and plasma levels are found.

Nitrosoureas- After intravenous infusion of 60 to 170 mg/m^2, peak plasma concentration of 5 micromolar is reached. Then, nitrosoureas decay with an initial half-life of 6 minutes and a second half-life of 68 minutes. The plasma clearance half-lives of the hydroxy-CCNU metabolites vary from 1 to 3 hours between patients.

Busulfan- Because of its insolubility in aqueous solutions, busulfan was available only as an oral preparation, previously. Later, an intravenous preparation was produced. Busulfan is widely used at a dose of 1 mg/kg every 6 hours for 4 days for myeloablative therapy prior to bone marrow transplantation. After a 1 mg/kg dose in adults and older children, there is a considerable variation in bioavailability, with peak plasma levels of 1 to 10 micromolar and elimination half-times between 1 and 7 hours. However, in young children (age 1–3), the peak plasma concentrations are less (1–5 micromolar), the mean elimination time is approximately 40% faster, and the AUC consistently less at 6 to 17 micromolar. All patients exhibit the AUCs of busulfan greater than one standard deviation from the mean values are under a very high risk of veno-occlusive disease of the liver [2, 4].

Hematopoietic Toxicity

In general, the clinical dose-limiting toxicity of alkylating agents is hematopoietic toxicity, particularly suppression of granulocytes and platelets. The nadir of granulocyte depression after alkylating agents is usually 8 to 16 days, and the granulocyte level usually return to normal within 20 days after a single dose of the agent [4]. Cyclophosphamide and ifosfamide are less hematopoietically toxic than other alkylating agents; granulocyte levels return to normal more rapidly, platelets are affected less, and repeated doses of cyclophosphamide and ifosfamide do not produce cumulative damage and progressive deterioration of the hematopoietic elements. In contrast, the nitrosoureas produce severe hematopoietic toxicity, with a delayed onset and nadirs of granulocytes and platelets occurring as late as 45 days. Busulfan also produces severe hematopoietic depression, with a selectivity for early myeloid precursors. The degree and duration of granulocyte depression after antitumor drug administration can be reduced by concomitant use growth factors [50]. Currently, growth factors that may stimulate the proliferation and restoration of megakaryocytes and platelets are also used [51].

Gastrointestinal Toxicity

Damage to the gastrointestinal tract is a toxicity that frequently occurs with high-dose regimens. Mucositis, stomatitis, esophagitis, and diarrhea occur with the use of high doses of alkylating agents and in particular after high doses of melphalan and thiotepa or combinations of alkylating agents including melphalan or thiotepa [52]. Significant mucositis is unusual even after very high doses of cyclophosphamide or ifosfamide. This lack of gastrointestinal toxicity is probably due to the presence of the enzyme aldehyde dehydrogenase in the epithelial cells of the gastrointestinal tract.

Nausea and vomiting are frequent side effects of alkylating agents. Although these side effects are not usually life threatening, they are major discomforts to patients and may result in the delay or discontinuation of therapy. The nausea and vomiting are mediated through the CNS and are not due to direct gastrointestinal toxicity. These effects are variable between patients. The frequency of nausea and vomiting increase when the dose of alkylating agents is increased.

Veno-Occlusive Disease of the Liver

This syndrome is characterized clinically by hepatomegaly, right upper quadrant pain, jaundice, ascites, and a high mortality rate from hepatic failure. Pathologically, the syndrome is associated with subendothelial thickening and narrowing of the hepatic venule lumen [53]. This complication is observed in about 25% of patients receiving high-dose cyclophosphamide and busulfan or cyclophosphamide and total body irradiation prior to allogeneic or autologous bone marrow transplantation for leukemia or lymphoma, and is also seen after other high-dose alkylating agent therapy.

Gonadal Damage

A serious toxicity of the alkylating agents is gonadal damage. It was first described in 1948 in patients treated with mechlorethamine [54]. After that, it was observed with the usage of other alkylating agents. Gonadal damage frequently results in aspermia or oligospermia in men treated with drug combinations including alkylating agents [55]. However, spermatogenesis and fertility may return after several years [56].

Amenorrhea associated with disappearance of mature and primordial ovarian follicles is determined in women treated with alkylating agents [57, 58]. The frequency of amenorrhea increases with the age of the woman and is more likely to be irreversible in older ages.

Pulmonary Damage

Pulmonary damage in the form of interstitial pneumonitis and fibrosis is associated with almost all of the alkylating anti-tumor drugs. It is presumably due to direct toxicity of the alkylating agents to pulmonary epithelial cells. The typical presentation is the onset of a nonproductive cough and dyspnea, which may progress to tachypnea and cyanosis and even to severe pulmonary insufficiency and death. This complication was first described in association with busulfan therapy [59], but subsequently it was described after cyclophosphamide [60], nitrosoureas [61], melphalan [62], chlorambucil [63], and mitomycin C [64] therapy.

Hemorrhagic Cystitis

The oxazophosphorines, cyclophosphamide and ifosfamide, produce bladder toxicity, which is not seen with other alkylating agents. This toxicity is a hemorrhagic cystitis, which may progress to massive hemorrhage [65]. The toxicity appears due to metabolites of these drugs, which are excreted into the urine. The metabolite principally responsible for this toxicity is acrolein [66]. Hemorrhagic cystitis is seen more commonly after ifosfamide therapy than cyclophosphamide, partly because higher doses of this agent are used. Renal tubular damage appearing with azotemia and elevated serum creatinine are also seen after ifosfamide.

The systemic administration of thiols can prevent or ameliorate the bladder damage derived from cyclophosphamide and ifosfamide, as the thiols inhibits conjugatation of aldehyde groups of acrolein and chloracetaldehyde. The most widely used compound to prevent oxazophosphorine mediated-bladder toxicity is the sodium salt of 2-mercaptoethane sulfonate (MESNA) [67]. MESNA is usually administered to all patients receiving ifosfamide and to patients who are receiving high-dose cyclophosphamide. Subclinical renal toxicity has been observed in children receiving ifosfamide despite MESNA administration [68], so that administration of MESNA does not eliminate the need for adequate hydration and careful observation of the patient.

Antidiuresis

An antidiuretic effect is commonly seen in patients receiving doses of cyclophosphamide of 50 mg/kg or greater [69]. This syndrome is characterized by a decrease in urine output 6 to 8 hours after drug administration, weight gain, a marked increase in urine osmolality, and a decrease in serum osmolality and sodium concentration.

Pericardial and pleural effusions may be seen, and seizures due to hyponatremia occurs after cyclophosphamide therapy, especially if low-sodium replacement fluids are administered. This antidiuretic syndrome appears to be due to an effect of cyclophosphamide metabolites on the distal renal tubule and is self-limited, with the excess fluid excreted over a period of about 12 hours. Administration of furosemide promotes free water clearance and ameliorate the syndrome [70].

Renal Toxicity

Renal toxicity is a serious toxicity of the nitrosoureas [71]. This effect is dose-related and may produce severe renal failure and death after administration of more than 1,200 mg of BCNU. Elevation of serum creatinine and other clinical evidences of renal toxicity may not be seen until after the completion of therapy. The histology of the kidneys in patients with renal nitrosourea damage is similar to that in radiation nephritis.

Alopecia

Although the association between an alkylating agent and alopecia was first described with busulfan therapy, this toxicity is predominantly associated with cyclophosphamide and ifosfamide therapy. The alopecia produced by these agents may be quite severe, especially if the agent is given in combination with vincristine or doxorubicin. Regrowth of the hair occurs after cessation of therapy and may be associated with a change in the texture and color of the hair. This toxicity is due to the entry of lipophilic metabolites into the hair follicles [72].

Allergic and Hypersensitivity Reactions

Since the alkylating agents react with many biologic molecules, it is not surprising that they would serve as haptenes and produce allergic reactions. The most frequent reactions reported so far are cutaneous hypersensitivities. Anaphylactic reactions are rare, but they are detected [73]. Patterns of cross-reactivity was not carefully defined, but cross-reactivity between agents of similar structure, such as the nitrogen mustards, were described.

Cardiotoxicity

The nonhematologic dose-limiting toxicity of cyclophosphamide is cardiac toxicity [74]. The fulminant syndrome is most frequently seen in patients receiving a total dose of cyclophosphamide greater than 200 mg/kg preparatory to bone marrow transplantation. The clinical course of the syndrome is the rapid onset of severe heart failure which is fatal within 10 to 14 days. The heart of such patients is dilated with patchy transmural hemorrhage and pericardial effusion. The microscopic findings are interstitial hemorrhage and edema, myocardial necrosis and vacuolar changes, and specific changes in the intramural small coronary vessels. Decreased electrocardiographic voltage and a transient increase in heart size are seen in high-dose cyclophosphamide receiving patients despite no apparent clinical symptoms, and the characteristic pathologic findings are present in such patients who die because of other causes. Cardiotoxicity and cardiomegaly are seen in patients receiving lower doses of cyclophosphamide in combination with other alkylating agents. Age greater than 50 years and previous adriamycin exposure appear to increase the risk of cyclophosphamide cardiotoxicity.

Neurotoxicity

In preclinical studies of alkylating agents, convulsions are often seen [75, 76]. At usual clinical doses of these agents, frank neurotoxicity is not usually seen but drowsiness and alterations of consciousness can be observed [77]. With higher doses and combinations of the alkylating agents, more clinical neurotoxicity is observed. At BCNU doses of 1,200 mg/m^2, severe CNS toxicity appears [78]. Intracarotid administration of BCNU causes blindness [79]. High-dose busulfan therapy produces seizures, and anticonvulsants are often used prophylactically in these patients [80].

Teratogenecity

Studies carried out in vivo and in embryo cultures demonstrated that virtually all of the alkylating agents are teratogenic [81]. The teratogenic effect is probably due to cytotoxic effects on the embryo by the same mechanisms by which the compounds are toxic to tumor cells. The available clinical information indicates that there is a definite risk of a malformed infant if the mother is treated with an alkylating agent during the first trimester of pregnancy [82, 83]. It has been shown that in a group consisting of 25 women who had received alkylating agents during the first trimester of pregnancy, fetal malformations have been determined in 4 of the women [84]. However, the administration of alkylation agents during the second and third trimesters is not associated with an increased risk of fetal malformation [85]. According to very recent data, the use of cytotoxic drugs during the first trimester to treat hematologic malignancies seems to be beneficial to both the mother and fetus, and chemotherapy during the first trimester can be considered if the cure of the patient is the goal [86]. It was shown that children of cancer survivors have not at significantly increased risk for congenital anomalies stemming from their parent's exposure to mutagenic cancer treatments [87].

Carcinogenesis

Since the initial reports of acute leukemia occurring in patients treated with alkylating agents [88-90], it has become increasingly obvious that this type of oncogenesis is a significant complication of alkylating agent therapy. Several studies have revealed that the rate of acute leukemia after alkylating agent therapy may be 10% or higher in certain groups of patients. Procarbazine and other methylating agents appear to be the most potent oncogenic agents, and melphalan appears to produce a higher rate of acute leukemia than cyclophosphamide [91]. The lesser leukemogenic potential of cyclophosphamide may well be related to the hematopoietic stem cell sparing effect of this agent. An increased rate of solid tumors has also been detected in patients treated with alkylating agents [92, 93]. Although sufficient data are not yet available to be certain, it seems that high-dose alkylating agent therapy administered in intermittent pulses relatively short period is less oncogenic than prolonged alkylating agent therapy.

Immunosuppression

Cyclophosphamide is particularly immunosuppressive [94] and is used for the treatment of autoimmune diseases. Cyclophosphamide is also used in preparative regimens for allogeneic transplantation due to its immunoablative activity. Low doses of cyclophosphamide and melphalan can enhance the immune response by selectively inhibiting the immune suppressor cells. Due to this effect, moderate doses of cyclophosphamide is used in conjunction with immunotherapy and biologic response modifiers, such as interleukin-2 [95].

The clinical significance of the immunosuppression produced by alkylating agents in their role as antitumor agents is not certain. The two major concerns are susceptibility to infection in the immunosuppressed host and the potential interference with a host immune response to the tumor. The available evidence indicate that most intermittent antitumor regimens do not produce a profound or prolonged immunosuppression [4].

Platinum Antitumor Compounds

The platinum antitumor agents are complexes of platinum with ligands that can be displaced by nucleophilic (electron-rich) atoms to form strong bonds with covalent characteristic. Thus, like the alkylating agents, the platinum agents form strong chemical bonds with thiol sulfurs and amino nitrogens in proteins and nucleic acids. Cisplatin went into clinical trials in the early 1970s [96] and was found to have significant antitumor activity against testicular cancer, lymphoma, squamous cell carcinoma of the head and neck, ovarian cancer, and bladder cancer. Because of its significant therapeutic effect in these tumors and activity against a number of other solid tumors, it became the most frequently used antitumor agent. Because of the renal toxicity and neurotoxicity of cisplatin, intensive efforts made to devise analogues with fewer of these toxicities. Extensive works led to development of carboplatin, which causes primarily hematopoietic toxicity and appears to have an antitumor effect similar to cisplatin [97] against the tumors. There is no evidence for cross-resistance between these two agents. A number of other platinum compounds are currently under investigation and are discussed below. The platinum compounds that are active antitumor agents can have either four or six ligands with a square planar or hexahedral configuration, respectively. Those which have four ligands have an oxidation state of +2, and those with six ligands have an oxidation state of +4. The chloride ligands of cisplatin and the other complexes with the 12 oxidation states can be exchanged for nucleophilic atoms in the biologic milieu, including the nitrogens of the DNA bases. If the chloride leaving ligands are replaced with carboxyl ester groups, as in carboplatin and oxaliplatin, higher concentrations are needed for cytotoxicity. The decreased renal and neurologic toxicity of these compounds are also probably due to the fact that they are less chemically reactive than cisplatin. Although there is considerable evidence that the formation of DNA adducts is responsible for the cytotoxicity of the platinum antitumor agents, the mechanisms involved in cytotoxicity are not well understood. Evidences are presented that the platinum adducts inhibit replication [98]. Heiger-Bernays and colleagues [99] demonstrated that as few as two platinum adducts per genome is sufficient for inhibition of DNA replication by cisplatin. A correlation between cytotoxicity of cisplatin and the duration of arrest in the G2 phase of the cell cycle was found by Sorenson and Eastman [100].

Oxaliplatin is similar to tetraplatin in its preclinical toxicity [101]. However, this compound is shown promising activity in gastrointestinal tumors, especially in combination with 5-FU and leucovorin. Oxaliplatin also demonstrates significant activity in patients with ovarian cancer who are previously received cisplatin [102]. Oxaliplatin demonstrates a modest effect (15% PR) in advanced, cisplatin-resistant non-small-cell lung patients [103].

A lipid-soluble platinum compound, JM216 (satraplatin), which can be administered orally evaluated clinically [104]. The new platinum analogues may not be totally cross-resistant with cisplatin due to differences in either cellular uptake or cellular detoxification [2, 4]. Decreased creatinine clearance results in higher plasma levels of both cisplatin and carboplatin, and potentially greater toxicity. After bolus administration of 100 mg/m^2 of cisplatin, initial peak plasma concentration of 3 to >5 microgram/ml ise achieved [105] with decreasing to less than 0.2 microgram/ml at 2 hours. After the usual clinical dose of about 300 mg/m^2 of carboplatin, peak plasma level of about 30 microgram/ml is reached, declining to about 5 microgram/ml at 2 hours. In typical clinical use, usually in combination with other agents, the platinum antitumor agents are given intravenously, either as a single dose or daily for several days, with repeated courses at 3 to 4 weeks. The agents are given as an infusion over several hours rather than as a bolus dose and, especially with very high doses, may be given as 24-hour or longer infusions. Due to the close relationships between plasma AUC of carboplatin and renal function, and between AUC of carboplatin and toxicity, dosing algorithms based on renal function were established and are now widely used in the dosing of carboplatin [106].

Cisplatin and carboplatin are also administered regionally. There are considerable experience with the intraperitoneal route, particularly in the treatment of ovarian cancer [107]. Very high intraperitoneal concentrations can be obtained, and systemic toxicities can be reduced by the concomitant systemic administration of thiosulfate [108]. Cisplatin are administered intra-arterially for the treatment of tumors in the extremities [109], brain tumors [110], carcinoma of the head and neck [111], carcinoma of the liver [112], and carcinoma of the bladder [113]. Cisplatin are also instilled into the pericardial sac for the treatment of malignant pericardial effusions [114].

Toxicities of Platinum Antitumor Compounds

Renal Toxicity

The most serious, and usually dose-limiting, toxicity of cisplatin is renal [4]. This toxicity is manifested clinically by elevated blood urine nitrogen (BUN) and creatinine. Toxicity is cumulative with continued cisplatin exposure, and is potentiated by other nephrotoxins. Decreases in serum electrolytes are associated with platinum renal toxicity, including symptomatic hypomagnesemia [115]. Although the toxicity may remain subclinical, or the renal function may return to normal, significant pathologic damage appears to persist. The pathology of the renal damage involves focal acute tubular necrosis, dilatation of convoluted tubules, thickened tubular basement membranes, formation of casts, and epithelial atypia of the collecting ducts [116]. High fluid intake with forced diuresis can reduce the incidence and severity of the renal toxicity. Systemic administration of thiols can reduce renal toxicity of cisplatin in animal models, and in a clinical trial, systemic diethyldithiodicarbamate appeared to reduce nephrotoxicity without affecting ototoxicity or myelosuppression. The nephrotoxicity of the second-generation platinum complexes, such as carboplatin and iproplatin, is markedly less than that of cisplatin.

Ototoxicity

Ototoxicity is a significant problem of cisplatin. This toxicity is characterized by tinnitus and hearing loss [117]. The hearing loss is usually in the high-frequency range, 4,000 to 8,000 Hz, but may occur in the lower ranges including the speech frequencies. Since the higher frequencies are usually involved, the hearing loss may not be symptomatic. The ototoxicity of cisplatin is dose- dependent and is usually cumulative with subsequent courses of the agent. Radiation prior to or simultaneous with the cisplatin administration enhances the toxicity [118], but this additive effect may be less if the cisplatin precedes the radiation [119]. The pathologic findings associated with ototoxicity in both experimental animals and patients are selective damage to the outer hair cells of the cochlea and lesions in the organ of Corti, the spiral ganglion and cochlear nerve, and the stria vascularis [120]. In studies of organ cultures of the cochlear structures, the hair cells are very sensitive to very low concentrations of cisplatin. Vestibular toxicity does not usually occur but can be seen. Vestibular toxicity is associated with degeneration of the maculae and cristae [121].

Neurotoxicity

The neurotoxicity observed with the administration of cisplatin consists principally of peripheral neuropathy involving both the upper and lower extremities, with paresthesias, weakness, tremors, and loss of taste. Seizures and leucoencephalopathy were also described [75, 76]. The neurotoxicity may be persistent and may progress after cessation of cisplatin therapy. Particularly severe neurotoxicity has been reported after intra-arterial infusions of cisplatin, with cranial nerve paralysis occurring after intra-arterial infusions for head and neck cancer, and severe peripheral neuropathy has been determined after lower limb perfusion. The neurotoxicity of ifosfamide has been reported to be enhanced by prior treatment with cisplatin. Since various pharmacologic maneuvers are able to control or reduce the nephrotoxicity and severe nausea and vomiting, neurotoxicity is the dose-limiting toxicity of cisplatin. An interesting observation is that treatment of animals with an ACTH analogue prevents cisplatin-mediated neurotoxicity and facilitates the recovery of established neurotoxicity but does not interfere with the antitumor effect of the agent. In a randomized, placebo-controlled clinical trial, ACTH analogue appeared to prevent or ameliorate the neurotoxicity of cisplatin [122].

Gastrointestinal Toxicity

Severe nausea and vomiting are significant problems of cisplatin appearing in almost all patients receiving the drug [4]. The cause of this toxicity is not firmly established. A study in animal model revealed that abdominal visceral innervation and 5-hydroxytryptamine receptors on visceral afferent nerves play a role in development of gastrointestinal toxicity. However, there is also evidence indicating the role of the chemoreceptor trigger zone in the medulla. The use of a dopamine antagonist, metoclopramide, prior to and during cisplatin administration is effective in controlling this toxicity, and the steroids dexamethasone or methylprednisolone alone or in combination with metoclopramide are also useful. More recently, antiserotonin analogues such as ondansetron and granisetron were proven highly effective in controlling nausea and vomiting after platinum administration. The gastrointestinal toxicities of carboplatin and iproplatin are much less than those of cisplatin.

Immune Effects

Although many of alkylating agents are significantly immunosuppressive, cisplatin appears to have no immunosuppressive effect at the usual clinical doses and may even augment immune function at these doses [4]. Monocyte-mediated cytotoxicity was found to be increased in ovarian cancer patients after cisplatin treatment.

Conclusion

All the studies provide strong evidence about effectivity of alkylating agents for treatment of all kinds of malignancies and even for relapsing tumors in children and adults.

References

[1]   Adair FE, Bagg HJ. Experimental and clinical studies on the treatment of cancer by dichloroethylsulfide (mustard gas). *Ann. Surg.* 1931; 93:190- 9.

[2]   Adamson PC, Bagatell R, Balis FM, Blaney SM. General principles of chemotherapy In: Pizzo Philip A, Poplack, David G. *Principles and*

practice of pediatric oncology. 6th ed. Hagerstown, MD: Lippincott Williams and Wilkins. pp 288-305.

[3]   Colvin M, Chabner BA. *Alkylating Agents in Cancer Chemotherapy: Principles and Practice.* Edited by BA Chabner, JM Collins. Philadelphia: Lippincott, 1990, pp 276–313.

[4]   Colvin M. Alkylating Agents and platinum anti-tumor compounds. In: Bast RCJr, Kufe DW, Pollack RE, et al. editors. *Holland-Frei Cancer Medicine*5th ed. Hamilton (ON): BC Decker; 2000. Bookshelf ID: NBK20984.

[5]   Goodman L S, Wintrobe M M, Dameshek W, Goodman J J. et al. Use of methyl-bis(beta-chlorethyl) amine hydrochloride for Hodgkins disease, lymphosarcoma, leukemia. *JAMA.* 1946;132:126-32.

[6]   Jacobson LO, Spurr CL, Barron ESG. et al. Studies on the effect of methyl-bis(beta-chloroethyl)amine hydrochloride on neoplastic diseases and allied disorders of the hematopoietic system. *JAMA.* 1946; 132: 263-71.

[7]   Rhoads CP. Nitrogen mustards in treatment of neoplastic disease. *JAMA.* 1946; 131:656-8.

[8]   Alarcon R A, Meienhofer J. Formation of the cytotoxic aldehyde acrolein during the in vitro degradation of cyclophosphamide. *Nature New Biol.* 1971; 233:250–2.

[9]   Lee S M, Crowther D, Scarffe J H. et al. Cyclophosphamide decreases O6-alkylguanine-DNA alkyltransferase activity in peripheral lymphocytes of patients undergoing bone marrow transplantation. *Br. J. Cancer.* 1992; 66: 331–6.

[10] Friedman H S, Pegg A E, Johnson S P. et al. Modulation of cyclophosphamide activity by O-6-alkylguanine-DNA alkyltransferase. *Cancer Chemother. Pharmacol.* 1999; 43: 80–5.

[11] Russo JE, Hilton J, Colvin OM. The role of aldehyde dehydrogenase isoenzymes in cellular resistance to the alkylating agent cyclophosphamide. In *Enzymology and Molecular Biology of Carbonyl Metabolism,* vol 2. New York, Liss, 1989, p 65.

[12] Antman K H, Elias A, Ryan L. Ifosfamide and mesna: response and toxicity at standard- and high-dose schedules. *Semin. Oncol.* 1990; 17: 68-73.

[13] Loehrer P J Sr, Lauer R, Roth B J, Williams S D. et al. Salvage therapy in recurrent germ cell cancer: ifosfamide and cisplatin plus either vinblastine or etoposide. *Ann. Intern. Med.* 1988;109:540-6.

[14] Pratt C B, Douglass E C, Etcubanas E. et al. Clinical studies of ifosfamide/mesna at St. Jude Children's Research Hospital, 1983–1988. *Semin. Oncol.* 1989; 16(Suppl 3):51-5.

[15] Boddy A V, Cole M, Pearson A D J, Idle J R. The kinetics of the auto-induction ifosfamide metabolism during continuous infusion. Cancer Chemother Pharmacol. 1995; 36: 53-60.

[16] Colvin M. The comparative pharmacology of cyclophosphamide and ifosfamide. *Semin Oncol.* 1982; 9:2-7.

[17] Goren MP, Wright RK, Pratt CB, Pell FE. Dechlorethylation of ifosfamide and neurotoxicity. *Lancet.* 1986; 2: 1219-20.

[18] Barlogie B, Jagannath S, Dixon D O. et al. High-dose melphalan and granulocyte-macrophage colony-stimulating factor for refractory multiple myeloma. *Blood.* 1990; 76: 677-80.

[19] Young R C, Walton L A, Ellenberg S S. et al. Adjuvant therapy in stage I and stage II epithelial ovarian cancer. *N. Engl. J. Med.* 1990; 322: 1021-5.

[20] Rivkin S E, Green S, Metch B. et al. Adjuvant CMFVP versus melphalan for operable breast cancer with positive axillary nodes: 10-year results of a Southwest Oncology Group Study. *J. Clin. Oncol.* 1989; 7: 1229-38.

[21] Johnson TM. Treatment and management of chronic lymphocytic leukemia in the elderly: what the pharmacist clinician should know. *Consult. Pharm.* 2012;27: 274-85.

[22] Shireen R, Brennan D, Flannelly G, Fennelly D, Lenehan P, Foley M. Survival in women with ovarian cancer before and after the introduction of adjuvant paclitaxel; a 25-year, single institution review. *Ir. Med. J.* 2012; 105:47-50.

[23] Portlock C S, Fischer D S, Cadman E. et al. High-dose pulse chlorambucil in advanced, low-grade non-Hodgkin lymphoma. *Cancer Treat. Rep.* 1987;71: 1029-31.

[24] Gutin P H, Levi J A, Wiernik P H, Walker M D. Treatment of malignant meningeal disease with intrathecal thioTEPA: a phase II study. *Cancer Treat. Rep.* 1977;61: 885-7.

[25] Ng S F, Waxman D J. N,N',N"-triethylenethiophosphoramide (thio-TEPA) oxygenation by constitutive hepatic P450 enzymes and modulation of drug metabolism and clearance in vivo by P450-inducing agents. *Cancer Res.* 1991; 51: 2340-5.

[26] Hagen B. Pharmacokinetics of thio-TEPA and TEPA in the conventional dose-range and its correlation to myelosuppressive effects. *Cancer Chemother. Pharmacol.* 1991;27: 373-8.

[27] Menichetti E T, Silva R R, Tummarello D, Miseria S. et al. Etoposide and mitomycin-C in pretreated metastatic breast cancer. *Tumori.* 1989; 75: 473-4.

[28] Wils J, Bleiberg H. Current status of chemotherapy for gastric cancer. *Eur. J. Cancer Clin. Oncol.* 1989;25: 3-8.

[29] Falletta J M, Cushing B, Lauer S. et al. Phase I evaluation of diaziquone in childhood cancer. A Pediatric Oncology Group study. *Invest. New Drugs.* 1990; 8: 167.

[30] Zhang XY, Lian Yan X, Guo W, et al. Anticancer activity and mechanisms of diacetyldianhydrogalactitol on hepatoma QGY-7703 cells. *Anticancer Drugs.* 2009;20: 926-31.

[31] Mishra KK, Squire S, Lamborn K, et al. Phase II TPDCV protocol for pediatric low-grade hypothalamic/chiasmatic gliomas: 15-year update. *J. Neurooncol.* 2010; 100: 121-7.

[32] Pacheco D Y, Stratton N K, Gibson N W. Comparison of the mechanism of action of busulfan with hepsulfam, a new antileukemic agent, in the L1210 cell line. *Cancer Res.* 1989;49: 5108-11.

[33] Ohanian M, Cortes J, Kantarjian H, Jabbour E. Tyrosine kinase inhibitors in acute and chronic leukemias. *Expert Opin. Pharmacother.* 2012; 13: 927-38.

[34] Al-Seraihy A, Ayas M, Al-Nounou R, et al. Outcome of allogeneic stem cell transplantation with a conditioning regimen of busulfan, cyclophosphamide and low-dose etoposide for children with myelodysplastic syndrome. *Hematol. Oncol. Stem Cell Ther.* 2011;4: 121-5.

[35] Walker M D, Alexander E Jr, Hunt W E. et al. Evaluation of BCNU and/or radiotherapy in the treatment of anaplastic gliomas. A cooperative clinical trial. *J. Neurosurg.* 1978;49: 333-43.

[36] Bonadonna G, Valgussa P, Santoro A. et al. Hodgkin's disease: the Milan Cancer Institute experience with MOPP and ABVD. *Recent Results Cancer Res.* 1989;117:169-74.

[37] Levin VA, Silver P, Hannigan J. et al. Superiority of post-radiotherapy adjuvant chemotherapy with CCNU, procarbazine, and vincristine (PCV) over BCNU for anaplastic gliomas. *Int. J. Radiat. Oncol. Biol. Phys.* 1990;18: 321-4.

[38] Spagnolo F, Queirolo P. Upcoming strategies for the treatment of metastatic melanoma. *Arch. Dermatol. Res.* 2012 ; 304:177-84.

[39] Auerbach, SD. Nonclassic alkylating agents. In *Cancer Chemotherapy: Principles and Practice.* Edited by BA Chabner, JM Collins. Philadelphia: Lippincott, 1990, pp 314–28.

[40] Newlands ES, Foster T, Zaknoen S. Phase I study of temozolamide (TMZ) combined with procarbazine (PCB) in patients with gliomas. *Br. J. Cancer* 2003 21;89: 248-51.

[41] Sun J, Deng Y, Wang S, Cao J, Gao X, Dong X. Liposomes incorporating sodium deoxycholate for hexamethylmelamine (HMM) oral delivery: development, characterization, and in vivo evaluation. *Drug Deliv.* 2010;17: 164-70.

[42] Sladek N. Human aldehyde dehydrogenases: potential pathological, pharmacological, and toxicological impact. *J. Biochem. Mol. Toxicol.* 2003; 17:7-23. Review.

[43] Struck R F, Kirk M C, Mellett L B, El-Dareer S, Hill D L. Urinary metabolites of the antitumor agent cyclophosphamide. *Mol. Pharmacol.* 1971;7: 519-29.

[44] Humphrey R L, Kvols L K. The influence of renal insufficiency on cyclophosphamide-induced hematopoietic depression and recovery. *Proc. Am. Assoc. Cancer Res.* 1974;15: 84-7.

[45] Wagner T, Heydrich D, Jork T, Voelcker G, Hohorst H J. Comparative study on human pharmacokinetics of activated ifosfamide and cyclophosphamide by a modified fluorometric test. *J. Cancer Res. Clin. Oncol.* 1981;100: 95-104.

[46] Struck, RF, Alberts, DS, Horne K. et al. Plasma pharmacokinetics of cyclophosphamide and its cytotoxic metabolites after intravenous versus oral administration in a randomized, crossover, trial. *Cancer Res.* 1987;47: 2723-6.

[47] Alberts D S, Chang S Y, Chen H -S G, Larcom B J, Evans T L. Comparative pharmacokinetics of chlorambucil and melphalan in man. *Recent Results Cancer Res.* 1980;74: 124-31.

[48] Tattersall M H N, Weinberg A. Pharmacokinetics of melphalan following oral or intravenous administration in patients with malignant disease. *Eur. J. Cancer.* 1978;14: 507-13.

[49] Wadler S, Egorin M J, Zuhowski E G. et al. Phase I clinical and pharmacokinetic study of thiotepa administered intraperitoneally in patients with advanced malignancies. *J. Clin. Oncol.* 1989;7:132-9.

[50] Brandt S J, Peters W P, Atwater S K. et al. Effect of recombinant human granulocyte-macrophage colony-stimulating factor on hemotopoietic reconstitution after high-dose chemotherapy and autologous bone marrow transplantation. *N. Engl. J. Med.* 1988;318:869-76.

[51] Ikeda Y, Miyakawa Y. Development of thrombopoietin receptor agonists for clinical use. *J. Thromb. Haemost.* 2009;7 Suppl 1: 239-44. Review.

[52] Antman K, Eder J P, Elias A. et al. High-dose thiotepa alone and in combination regimens with bone marrow support. *Semin. Oncol.* 1990; 17(Suppl 3):33-8.

[53] Jones R J, Lee K S, Beschorner W E. et al. Venoocclusive disease of the liver following bone marrow transplantation. Transplantation. 1987;44: 778-92.

[54] Spitz S. The histological effects of nitrogen mustards on human tumors and tissues. *Cancer.* 1948;1:383-98.

[55] Sherins R J, DeVita V T. Effect of drug treatment for lymphoma on male reproductive capacity. *Ann. Intern. Med.* 1973;79: 216-20.

[56] Blake D B, Heller R H, Hsu S H, Schacter B Z. Return of fertility in a patient with cyclophosphamide-induced azoospermia. Johns Hopkins *Med J.* 1976; 139:20.

[57] Kyoma H, Wada T, Nishizawa T, Iwanaga T, Aoki Y. Cyclophosphamide-induced ovarian failure and its therapeutic significance in patients with breast cancer. *Cancer.* 1977;39: 1403-9.

[58] Cho WK, Lee JW, Chung NG, Jung MH, Cho B, Suh BK, et al. Primary ovarian dysfunction after hematopoietic stem cell transplantation during childhood: busulfan-based conditioning is a major concern. *J. Pediatr. Endocrinol. Metab.* 2011;24: 1031-5.

[59] Oliner H, Schwartz R, Rubio F Jr, Dameshek W. Interstitial pulmonary fibrosis following busulfan therapy. *Am. J. Med.* 1961;31: 134-9.

[60] Wiedrich T, Keller D, Arya S, Gilbert E, Trigg M. Adverse histopathologic effects of chemotherapeutic agents in childhood leukemia and lymphoma. *Pediatr. Pathol.* 1984;2: 267-83.

[61] Bailey C C, Marsden H B, Jones P H. Fatal pulmonary fibrosis following 1,3-bis (2-chloroethyl)-1-nitrosourea (BCNU) therapy. *Cancer. 1978*;42: 74-7.

[62] Codling B W, Chakera T M. Pulmonary fibrosis following therapy with melphalan for multiple myeloma. *J. Clin. Pathol.* 1972;25: 668-73.

[63] Cole R C, Myers T J, Klatsky A U. Pulmonary disease with chlorambucil therapy. *Cancer.* 1978;41: 455-9.

[64] Orwoll E S, Kiessling P J, Patterson J R. Interstitial pneumonia from mitomycin. *Ann. Intern. Med.* 1978; 89: 35-5.

[65] Philips F S, Sternberg S S, Cronin A P, Vidal P M. Cyclophosphamide and urinary bladder toxicity. *Cancer Res.* 1961; 21: 1577-89.

[66] Cox P J. Cyclophosphamide cystitis-identification of acrolein as the causative agent. *Biochem. Pharmacol.* 1979; 28: 2045-9.

[67] Brock N. The development of mesna for the inhibition of urotoxic side effects of cyclophosphamide, ifosfamide, and other oxazaphosphorine cytostatics. *Recent Results Cancer Res.* 1980; 74:270-7.

[68] Pratt C B, Horowitz M E, Meyer W H. et al. Phase II trial of ifosfamide in children with malignant solid tumors. *Cancer Treat. Rep.* 1987; 71:131.

[69] Bode U, Seif S M, Levine A A. Studies on the antidiuretic effect of cyclophosphamide: vasopressin release and sodium excretion. *Med. Pediatr. Oncol.* 1980;8: 295-303.

[70] Green T P, Mirkin B L. Prevention of cyclophosphamide-induced antidiuresis by furosemide infusion. *Clin. Pharmacol. Ther.* 1981; 29: 634-42.

[71] Harmon W E, Cohen H J, Schneeberger E E, Grupe W E. Chronic renal failure in children treated with methyl CCNU. *N. Engl. J. Med.* 1979; 300:1200-3.

[72] Feil V S, Lamoureaux C J H. Alopecia activity of cyclophosphamide metabolites and related compounds in sheep. *Cancer Res.* 1974; 34: 2596-8.

[73] Weiss RB, Bruno S. Hypersensitivity reactions to cancer chemotherapeutic agents. *Ann. Intern. Med.* 1981; 94:66-72.

[74] Steinherz L J, Steinherz P G. Cyclophosphamide cardiotoxicity. *Cancer Bull.* 1985; 37:231.

[75] Newton HB. Neurological complications of chemotherapy to the central nervous system. *Handb. Clin. Neurol.* 2012;105:903-16.

[76] Marosi C.Complications of chemotherapy in neuro-oncology. *Handb. Clin. Neurol.* 2012;105:873-85.

[77] Bethlenfalvay N C, Bergin J J. Severe cerebral toxicity after intravenous nitrogen mustard therapy. *Cancer.* 1972;29: 366-72.

[78] Takvorian T, Parker L M, Hochberg F H. et al. Single high-dose of BCNU with autologous bone marrow (ABM). *Proc. AACR Am. Soc. Clin. Oncol.* 1980; 21: 341-6.

[79] Yamada K, Bremer A M, West C R. et al. Intra-arterial BCNU therapy in the treatment of metastatic brain tumor from lung carcinoma. *Cancer.* 1979; 44: 2000-7.

[80] Vassal G, Deroussent A, Hartmann O. et al. Dose-dependent neurotoxicity of high-dose-busulfan in children: a clinical and pharmacological study. *Cancer Res.* 1990;50: 6203-7.

[81] Gibson J E, Becker B A. Teratogenicity of structural truncates of cyclophosphamide in mice. *Teratology.* 1971;4:141-7.

[82] Mirkes P E. Cyclophosphamide teratogenesis: a review. *Teratog. Carcinog. Mutagen.* 1985; 5: 75-88.

[83] Garrett M J. Teratogenic effects of combination chemotherapy. *Ann. Intern. Med.* 1974; 80: 667.

[84] Nicholson H O. Cytotoxic drugs in pregnancy. *J. Obstet. Gynaecol. Br. Common.* 1968; 75: 307-12.

[85] Ortega J. Multiple agent chemotherapy including bleomycin of non-Hodgkin's lymphoma during pregnancy. *Cancer.* 1977;40: 2829-34.

[86] Avilés A, Neri N, Nambo MJ. Hematological malignancies and pregnancy: Treat or no treat during first trimester. *Int. J. Cancer.* 2012 Apr 18. doi: 10.1002/ijc.27560.

[87] Signorello LB, Mulvihill JJ, Green DM, et al. Congenital anomalies in the children of cancer survivors: a report from the childhood cancer survivor study. *J. Clin. Oncol.* 2012; 30: 239-45.

[88] Reimer R R, Hoover R, Fraumeni J F Jr, Young R C. Acute leukemia after alkylating-agent therapy of ovarian cancer. *N. Engl. J. Med.* 1977; 297:177-81.

[89] Tucker M A, Coleman C N, Cox R S, Varghese A, Rosenberg S A. Risk of second cancers after treatment for Hodgkins disease. *N. Engl. J. Med.* 1988; 318: 76-81.

[90] Dorr F A, Coltman C A Jr. Second cancers following antineoplastic therapy. *Curr. Probl. Cancer.* 1985;9: 1-43.

[91] Green M H, Harris E L, Gershenson D M. et al. Melphalan may be a more potent leukemogen than cyclophosphamide. *Ann. Intern. Med.* 1986; 105:360-7.

[92] Penn I. Second malignant neoplasm associated with immunosuppressive medications. *Cancer.* 1976;37: 1024-32.

[93] Braam KI, Overbeek A, Kaspers GJ, etal. Malignant melanoma as second malignant neoplasm in long-term childhood cancer survivors: A systematic review. *Pediatr. Blood Cancer.* 2012 Jan 9. doi: 10.1002/ pbc.24023. [Epub ahead of print].

[94] Makinodan T, Santos G W, Quinn R P. Immunosuppressive drugs. *Pharmacol. Rev.* 1970;22: 189-247.

[95] Mitchell M S, Kempf R A, Harel W. et al. Effectiveness and tolerability of low-dose cyclophosphamide and low-dose intravenous interleukin-2 in disseminated melanoma. *J. Clin. Oncol.* 1988;6: 409-24.

[96] Lippman A J, Helson C, Helson L, Krakoff I H. Clinical trials of cis-diamminedichloroplatinum (NSC-119875). *Cancer Chemother. Rep.* 1973; 57: 191-200.

[97] Skarlos D V, Samantas E, Kosmidis P. et al. Randomized comparison of etoposide-cisplatin vs. etoposide-carboplatin and irradiation in small-cell lung cancer. A Hellenic Cooperative Oncology Group Study. *Ann. Oncol.* 1994; 5: 601-7.

[98] Pinto A L, Lippard S J. Sequence-dependent termination of in vitro DNA synthesis by cis- and trans-diamminedichloroplatinum(II). *Proc. Natl. Acad. Sci. U S A.* 1985;82: 4616-9.

[99] Heiger-Bernays W J, Essigmann J M, Lippard S J. Effect of the antitumor drug cis-diamminedichloroplatinum(II) and related platinum complexes on eukaryotic DNA replication. *Biochemistry.* 1990; 29: 8461-8.

[100] Sorenson C M, Eastman A. Influence of cis-diammine-dichloroplatinum(II) on DNA synthesis and cell cycle progression in excision repair proficient and deficient Chinese hamster ovary cells. *Cancer Res.* 1988; 48:6703-7.

[101] Extra J M, Espie M, Calvo F. et al. Phase I study of oxaliplatin in patients with advanced cancer. *Cancer Chemother. Pharmacol.* 1990; 25: 299-303.

[102] Sessa C, Huinink W W T, du Bois A. Oxaliplatin in ovarian cancer. *Ann. Oncol.* 1999; 10: 55–7.

[103] Jiang L, Yang KH, Guan QL, Mi DH, Wang J. Cisplatin plus etoposide versus other platin-based regimens for patients with extensive small cell lung cancer: a systematic review and meta analysis of randomized controlled trials. *Intern. Med. J.* 2012 Apr 25. doi: 10.1111/j.1445-5994.2012.02821.

[104] Kelland L R, Abel G, MeKeage M J. et al. Preclinical antitumor evaluation of bis-acetato-ammine-dichloro-cyclohexylamine platinum (IV): an orally active platinum drug. *Cancer Res.* 1993; 53:2581-6.

[105] Himmelstein KJ, Patton TF, Belt RJ, Taylor S, Repta AJ, Sternson LA. Clinical kinetics on intact cisplatin and some related species. *Clin. Pharmacol. Ther.* 1981 ; 29:658-64.

[106] Calvert, H, Judson I, van der Vijgh W J. Platinum complexes in cancer medicine: pharmacokinetics and pharmacodynamics in relation to toxicity and therapeutic activity. *Cancer Surv.* 1993;17: 189-98.

[107] Speyer J L, Beller U, Colombo N. et al. Intraperitoneal carboplatin: favorable results in women with minimal residual ovarian cancer after cisplatin therapy. *J. Clin. Oncol.* 1990;8: 1335-41.

[108] Markman M, Cleary S, Howell S B. Nephrotoxicity of high-dose intracavitary cisplatin with intravenous thiosulfate protection. *Eur. J. Cancer Clin. Oncol.* 1985; 21:101 -8.

[109] Bacci G, Picci P, Ruggieri P. et al. Primary chemotherapy and delayed surgery (neoadjuvant chemotherapy) for osteosarcoma of the extremities. The Instituto Rissoli Experience in 127 patients treated preoperatively with intravenous methotrexate (high versus moderate doses) and intra-arterial cisplatin. *Cancer.* 1990;65: 2539-53.

[110] Follezou J Y, Fauchon F, Chiras J. Intra-arterial infusion of carboplatin in the treatment of malignant gliomas: a phase II study. *Neoplasma.* 1989; 36: 349-52.

[111] Baker S R, Wheeler R. Intra-arterial chemotherapy for head and neck cancer. Part 2: clinical experience. *Head Neck Surg.* 1984;6: 751-9.

[112] Kasugai H, Kojima J, Tatsuta M. et al. Treatment of hepatocellular carcinoma by transcatheter arterial cisplatin and ethiodized oil. *Gastroenterology.* 1989; 97: 965-71.

[113] Jacobs S C, Menashe D S. Intra-arterial chemotherapy for bladder cancer. *Prog. Clin. Biol. Res.* 1990;350:101-6.

[114] Fiorentino M V, Daniele O, Morandi P. et al. Intrapericardial instillation of cis-platin in malignant pericardial effusion. *Cancer.* 1988; 62: 1904-6.

[115] Schilsky R L, Anderson T. Hypomagnesemia and renal magnesium wasting in patients receiving cisplatin. *Ann. Intern. Med.* 1979; 90: 929-31.

[116] Uehara T, Yamate J, Torii M, Maruyama T. Comparative nephrotoxicity of Cisplatin and nedaplatin: mechanisms and histopathological characteristics. *J. Toxicol. Pathol.* 2011 ;24:87-94.

[117] Skinner R, Pearson A D, Amineddine H A. et al. Ototoxity of cisplatinum in children and adolescents. *Br. J. Cancer.* 1990; 61: 927-31.

[118] Granowetter L, Rosenstock J G, Packer R J. Enhanced cis-platinum neurotoxicity in pediatric patients with brain tumors. *J. Neuro oncol.* 1983;1: 293-7.

[119] Kretschmar C S, Warren M P, Lavally B L. et al. Ototoxicity of preradiation cisplatin for children with central nervous system tumors. *J. Clin. Oncol.* 1990; 8: 1191-8.

[120] Boheim K, Bichler E. Cisplatin-induced ototoxicity: audiometric findings and experimental cochlear pathology. *Arch. Otorhinolaryngol.* 1985; 242:1-6.

[121] Wright C G, Schaefer S D. Inner ear histopathology in patients treated with cis-platinum. *Laryngoscope.* 1982; 92: 1408-13.

[122] van der Hoop R G, Vecht C J, van der Burg M E. et al. Prevention of cisplatin neurotoxicity with an ACTH(4-9) analogue in patients with ovarian cancer. *N. Engl. J. Med.* 1990; 322: 89-94.

In: Alkylating Agents …
Editor: Yildiz Dincer

ISBN: 978-1-62618-487-9
© 2013 Nova Science Publishers, Inc.

Chapter IV

Resistance Mechanisms for Alkylating Agent-Mediated Chemotherapy

*Ilhan Onaran**

Istanbul University Cerrahpasa Medical Faculty,
Department of Medical Biology, Istanbul, Turkey

Abstract

Despite significant advances in the treatment of cancer, resistance to chemotherapeutics is a major handicap that limits the effectiveness of anti-cancer drug treatment. Accumulating findings suggest that the mechanisms responsible for appearance of a drug-resistant phenotype are several, and contribute to the multifactorial nature of the problem. Resistance to alkylating agents at cellular level can occur via various mechanisms including increased drug efflux, drug inactivation, alterations in the ability of the cell to recognize and process alkylation adducts on DNA, and acquiring mechanisms to escape apoptosis. In addition to intracellular mechanisms, other contributing factors, such as the extracellular matrix and cancer stem cells, might be also involved in drug resistance. However, new findings indicating importance of epigenetic changes and microRNAs suggest that resistance against

* E-mail: ilonaran@istanbul.edu.tr

alkylating agents is much more complex than expected. In this chapter, previously described processes related to resistance to alkylating agents are reviewed and a few informative examples of the genetic basis of known biochemical mechanisms involved in resistance to alkylating agents are evaluated.

Introduction

Many cancer patients undergoing chemotherapy achieve a complete remission. Successful treatment of patients with certain malignancies indicate the high potential of current chemotherapeutic agents. Unfortunately, some patients are doomed to relapse and death due to failure of cancer therapy. There are multiple factors that determine tumor response to chemotherapy. One of the main factors is tumor resistance to drug treatment, which may be either regrowth of tumor after an initial response, a partial response, or a lack of response [1]. If an anticancer agent administered at maximal tolerated dose is unable to inhibit the tumor growth, this could be determined as complete tumor resistance. Based upon the clinical practice, drug resistance can be classified as either intrinsic (primary or innate) or acquired (secondary) in relation to the time of onset. However, types of resistance to alkylating agents as well as other chemotherapeutic drugs may also be classified in several ways, depending on pharmacodynamic, kinetic, genetic, tumor cell characteristics and factors in the tumor environment [2].

In intrinsic resistance, tumors do not respond from the outset and the resistance can occur at the beginning of the drug treatment in nearly 50% of all cancer cases. Non small cell lung cancer may be given as an example for intrinsic resistance. Nevertheless, in the acquired resistance, the tumor cells initially respond to therapy, but the resistance may develop after a period of time. Although the benefit of chemotherapy is clear for many patients, tumor recurrence develops in some patients just within 6–9 months after the treatment. Moreover, tumors that are resistant to one particular drug are either already cross-resistant or develop resistance to other chemotherapy drugs quickly. The knowledge about various resistance mechanisms to chemotherapy has increased over the years. as the result of a large number of tissue culture studies carried on drug resistant cell lines generated by continuous exposure of parental cells to chemotherapeutic agents. This increased knowledge revealed that various mechanisms are involved in drug resistance in given individuals. Resistance to alkylating agents as well as other chemotherapeutics can be envisioned at three levels; the level of the cell, the level of the tumor mass, and the level of the tumor /host interaction. Mechanisms of drug resistance have been intensively studied at the cellular level by using cell culture models which have the advantage of easy selection of resistant cells to a given cytotoxic agent. Meanwhile, microarray evaluation of alkylating agent-resistant cell lines from various tumors allowed the identification of genes that may be involved in resistance. Such studies have revealed a number of molecular mechanisms of drug resistance operative at cellular level. In addition, there are good evidences for a general agreement with mechanisms encountered clinically. Although all normal cells are alike in their response to drugs, cancer cells have a heterogeneity in response to therapy due to their own way. Functional gene mutations or other changes that affect the expression of genes encoding proteins that participate to drug response are important determinants of drug resistance. Accordingly, pointing to genetic and epigenetic mechanisms that modulate alkylating agent toxicity, the response of an individual to alkylating agents can vary considerably from tissue to tissue and from person to person. In addition to host factors, each tumor cell from a given patient can have a different genetic make-up, depending on the high frequency of dynamic mutation due to genomic instability in cells. Meanwhile, different random variations among the individual cells within a cancer may lead to an appearance of different tumor clones possessing various sensitivities to the action of administered anticancer agent. While cells within the tumor clone that are sensitive to anticancer agent die, resistant cells continue to proliferate.

Mechanisms of Resistance to Alkylating Agents

Although a single mechanism can occur in tumor cells for resistance to alkylating agents, theoretically, it is very rare in practice [3]. In some patients, prolonged exposure to a single drug may lead to the development of resistance to multiple structurally unrelated compounds, known as multidrug resistance (MDR). This type of resistance indicates the complexity of the problem. MDR can be derived from mutational (genetic) or nonmutational (epigenetic) processes in cancer cells. In genetic resistance, mutational changes leading to drug resistance appear to be simple point mutations or to be associated with extensive chromosomal changes or with gene amplification leading to overexpression of resistance factors. Nonmutational changes can arise due to aberrant methylation of cytidine phosphate guanosine (CpG) islands located at or near the promoters of critic genes. Although genetic and epigenetic processes are different mechanisms, they finally cause the same outcome, resistance to drugs. As respect with this fact, drug resistance is a multifactorial phenomenon and tumor cells become resistant to alkylating drugs by multiple interrelated or independent pathways. This phenomenon includes changes in cellular responses, such as increased cell ability to repair of damaged DNA, toleration to stress conditions and acquired mechanisms to escape from apoptosis. Cell behaviour against anticancer drugs leading to these final alterations are described in Figure I. As shown in Figure 1, recent studies suggest that these basic molecular mechanisms in tumour cells to anti-neoplastic chemotherapeutic alkylating agents; 1) a reduction in the uptake of the drug, 2) increased detoxification via interaction of the drug with intracellular thiols, 3) alterations in the ability of the cell to recognize and process alkylation adducts of DNA. As will be described in a later section, additional contributing factors, such as extracellular matrix might be also involved in drug resistance. However, this information alone could not explain the drug-resistant phenotype to alkylating agents.

These resistance mechanisms are cell line dependent so that a particular tumor may exhibit one, two or even all the above-mentioned mechanisms. In this chapter, previously described processes related to resistance to alkylating agents are discussed and a few informative examples of the genetic basis of known biochemical mechanisms involved in resistance to alkylating agents are evaluated.

Decreased Intracellular Accumulation of Alkylating Agents

Anticancer drugs must diffuse into tumour tissue and cells in a concentration sufficient to exert a therapeutic effect. The distribution of many anticancer drugs in tumour tissue is incomplete because of resistance of tumor cells to chemotherapy. In the level of a single cell, intracellular distribution of alkylating agents is a critical factor in the chemotherapy as cellular DNA is their target. Therefore, the mechanisms related to decrease of intracellular accumulation of anticancer drugs play an important role in the formation of drug resistance in tumor cells. However, it should be kept in mind *that drug accumulations alone do not provide a good indication of cytotoxic potencies.*

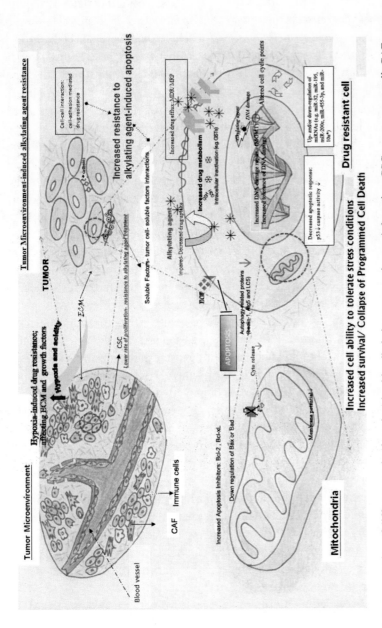

Figure 1. Representation of different mechanisms involved in alkylating agent resistance/adaptation. CSC: cancer stem cell; CAF: cancer associated fibroblast; EGF: epidermal growth factor; MGMT: O⁶-methylguanine DNA methyltransferase; Cyt c: Cytochrome c; glutathione: GSH; ↓: decrease; ↑ increase.

One of the suggested mechanisms for drug penetration deficiency through tumour cells *is decreased drug uptake and/or increased drug efflux. Several of alkylating drugs such as melphalan and* mechlorethamine enter cells through *active transport systems.* Reduced *active transport of* these drugs may be associated with tumor resistance. This mechanism was demonstrated in several alkylating agent-resistant tumor models [4]. CD98 is a heterodimeric membrane transport protein that preferentially transports drugs with branched-chain. In melphalan-resistant myeloma cells and mechlorethamine–resistant L51784 lymphoblast cells, down-regulation of CD98 is associated with reduced drug uptake.

Resistance may also have derived from increased alkylating agent efflux from cells or from nucleus into cytoplasm. In the frame of pharmacokinetic mechanisms, one of the factors responsible for resistance of tumor cells to alkylating and platinium agents includes acceleration of the efflux of these cytotoxic agent. Increased drug efflux lowers intracellular drug concentrations. However, as a result of multifactorial nature of the drug resistance, reduction in drug accumulation is not directly proportional to the degree of resistance.

The efflux system which plays a particularly significant role in the metabolism of drugs is an energy-dependent efflux pump. The GSH conjugates of a number of alkylating agents, including melphalan, cyclophosphamide, chlorambucil, and nitrogen mustards are the substrates of energy-dependent efflux pumps. It moves these conjugates which are more polar and less active than their parent compounds from inside of the cell to the outside decreasing their intra-cellular concentrations. The resistance to alkylating agents seen in some human tumors may be due to increased activity of the transport system in the cellular membrane.

According to the HUGO Gene Nomenclature Committee, membrane transporters were divided into two main families; the ATP binding cassette (ABC) transporter family and the solute carrier transporter family. In humans, ABC transporter family is relatively well characterized transporter as respect with its ability to transport drugs; and is considered as efflux pump of chemotherapeutic agents. Discussions about ABC transporters associated the resistance to alkylating agents are generally concentrated on MDR1/Pglycoprotein, and MRPs.

P-gp or also called multidrug resistance-1 (MDR1), encoded by the MDR-1/ABC1 gene, is the first identified mammalian multidrug transporter which is expressed in many healthy organs [5]. MDR1 expressed in normal tissue has physiologic functions specific to those tissues such as secretion of steroid hormones and excretion of natural toxic substances. Furthermore, it plays an important role in preventing the uptake of xenobiotics. MDR1 proteins function as a flippase for its substrates from the inner surface plasma membrane to the outer surface. ATP hydrolysis supplies the energy required for this active drug transport. The binding and subsequent hydrolysis of ATP by nucleotide-binding domain of MDR1 drive conformational changes that transport molecules across the membrane. MDR1 transports unmodified neutral or positively charged hydrophobic compounds. Meanwhile MDR1 is known to bind and transport over 200 pharmacological agents. Because of its high transport capacity and broad substrate recognition, it also plays an important role in development of drug resistance in tumor cells. It is known that MDR1 causes the development of drug resistance in a variety of cancer types derived from tissues with excretory or secretory function, such as colon, kidney, adrenocortical or hepatocellular carcinomas, as well as in some tumors which acquire resistance after chemotherapy including acute myeloid leukemia (AML), various childhood tumors and local regionally advanced breast cancer. MDR1 in these tumors is intrinsically over-expressed and well correlates with certain clinically observed drug resistance. Experimental studies with tumor cells grown in tissue culture show that expression or overexpression of MDR1 can be causative for chemoresistance [6]. Clinical studies, in agreement with the findings of the experimental studies, suggest that MDR1 regulates the pharmacokinetic of various types of clinically important drugs including classical alkylating agents and platinum analogues. After all, whether increased levels of MDR1 found in some alkylating agent-resistant tumors actually contribute to resistance is still a controversial issue.

The multidrug resistance-associated (MRP) gene family composed of at least eight members (MRP1–8) has been associated with cellular efflux of a variety of drugs [7]. However, only MRP1 and MRP2 (cMOAT) appears to be important in some alkylating agent-resistant tumor models. Resistance mediated by MRPs is similar to the pattern seen with MDR1-mediated chemoresistance. Increased MRP1 or MRP2 expression was detected in several cancer lines which are resistant to alkylating agents such as cisplatin and chlorambucil [8]. Their expression levels were also significantly increased in the relapsed patient group. However, cells transfected with MRP1 were not resistant to cisplatin, suggesting that this pump alone is not enough to confer resistance to platinum compounds [9].

It is not yet clear whether influx and efflux transporters play a clinically determinative role in the alkylating drug sensitivity and resistance of human tumours, because there are contrary findings for several pumps such as MRP1, MRP2, *MDR1* and lung resistance-related protein.

Intracellular Inactivation of Alkylating Agents

There are a number of enzyme systems within the cell that have the capacity to detoxify alkylating agents. One of the most important of these detoxification pathways is glutathione (GSH, γ-glutamyl-cysteinyl-glycine) system. Altered GSH metabolism in tumors was observed in many different human cancers [10, 11]. Alterations in the GSH metabolism were also observed in tumor cells resistant to alkylating agents. Along with the drug efflux system, GSH and its related enzymes potentiate tumor cells to resist against various cytotoxic drugs including alkylating agents such as melphalan, cyclophosphamide and chlorambucil. Currently, elevated intracellular GSH levels and the overexpression and/or unregulated activation of one or more of the GSH-related enzymes are thought to contribute to the development of tumor cell resistance to alkylating agents.

Glutathione, the most abundant thiol present in mammalian cells (up to 10 mM), plays pivotal roles in cell protection against free radicals, in nutrient metabolism, and in regulation of many cellular processes. As addition to these properties, GSH-associated metabolism is also a major mechanism for cellular protection against cancer-related risk factors that generate reactive oxygen species (ROS). The sulfhydryl group of cysteine in GSH can act either as a hydrogen bond donor or as an acceptor for various substrates. Above all, GSH forms conjugates with a variety of alkylating agents by Glutathione S-transferase (GST) dependent and non-enzymatic reactions. The conjugates are thought to be less toxic to cancerous cells as well as healthy *cells.* Melphalan, cyclophosphamide and chlorambucil are substrates for GSTs. Therefore, GSH may contribute to development of resistance to alkylating agents; especially this is valid for platinium analogues-induced cytotoxicity. Increases in cellular GSH concentration is correlated with increased resistance in a number of alkylating agent-resistant tumor models. Although contrary studies are also available, this is widely confirmed by clinical studies. Resistance due to elevated GSH is a reversible phenomenon. GSH depletion in human tumor cell lines which have high levels of GSH sensitizes cells to many cytotoxic compounds including alkylating agents (melphalan, nitrogen mustard, chlorambucil, cyclophosphamide, BCNU (N,N'-bis(2-chloroethyl)-N-nitrosourea) [12]. High intracellular level of GSH leads to increased conjugation of drugs and thus, inhibits the formation of the reactive alkylating moiety. Conjugation of the platinum analogues such as cisplatin and oxaliplatin by GSH may cause resistance because of the binding and subsequently blocking their action, enhancing DNA repair, or reducing cisplatin-induced oxidative stress [13].

GSH binding with cisplatin in the cytoplasm or with platinum-DNA monofunctional adducts in the nucleus can prevent the formation of potentially cytotoxic cross-links. Beyond this, glutathionyl-platinum complexes which are toxic, are known to be transported by various ATP-dependent efflux pumps [14]. As discussed above, ABC transporter proteins may transport GSH-platinum complexes out of the tumor cells, contributing to reduced intracellular drug accumulation.

In addition to changes in GSH levels, expression rate of GST is also important in development of resistance. Microarray analyses have shown that overexpression of GST in mammalian tumor cells may contribute to development of resistance to various anticancer agents and chemical carcinogens [15, 16].

Electrophilic alkylating agents can form conjugates with glutathione via glutathione S-transferases-mediated reactions as well as a non-enzymatic pathway. Glutathione S-transferases (EC 2.5.1.18) ubiquitously expressed in most living organisms are a superfamily of multifunctional, dimeric enzymes which catalyze the conjugation of GSH to generally hydrophobic and electrophilic compounds. Many carcinogens, therapeutic drugs such as alkylating agents and free radical generating anti-cancer drugs are the substrate for GST [17]. According to structure, substrate specificity, chemical affinity and the kinetic behavior of the enzyme, at least seven different classes (alpha, mu, pi, theta, zeta, omega, and sigma) of soluble GSTs were identified so far. The GST enzyme family in mammals includes the cytosolic isoforms GST-alpha (GSTA), mu (GSTM), pi (GSTP), theta (GSTT) and sigma (GSTS). The major enzymes involved in intracellular inactivation of alkylating agents are GST-alpha and GSTpi. One of the distinctive properties of GST-mediated detoxification systems is their capacity to recognize diverse chemical structures. Although multiple GSTs recognize many anticancer drugs as substrate, specific isoenzymes of the GSTs have a preferential substrate specificity. For example, even though GSTT1, GSTM2, and GSTM3 have BCNU conjugating activity, GSTT1 exhibits 14-fold higher GST-BCNU conjugating activity than other isotypes [18]. However, it was also reported that drug resistance to alkylating agents is primarily derived from high expression levels of GSTs rather than their substrate affinity [19]. The majority of human tumor cell lines selected as resistant to alkylating agents overexpress GSTP1 [12]. It was shown by experimental studies that the transfection of GST Pi subclass in human carcinoma cells induces in vitro resistance to cisplatin and melphalan. In addition, there is also an evidence that glutathione transferase omega 1-1 (GSTO1-1) overexpression may play an anti-apoptotic role in cell resistance to cisplatin toxicity [20].

In spite of a weak interaction between GSTP1-1 and the majority of anticancer drugs, increased expression of this isotype was found to be correlated with the development of the multidrug-resistant phenotype. GST-Pi was shown to be overexpressed in many cancer tissues such as breast, colon, kidney, lung, and ovary as well as in drug resistant cell lines. This data revealed that elevated GST-Pi expression may be of direct relevance both to acquired resistance and in natural resistance. Moreover, high GSTP1 expression in many solid tumors and leukemias was associated with resistance to drugs including alkylating agents, failure of therapy and poor patient survival [21]. Analysis of gene expression in tumor cells from patients with cisplatin-resistant cancer revealed that the increased expression of GSTP1 together with elevated GSH significantly contributes to the resistant phenotype at clinical level [22].

Interindividual differences in resistance development may be attributed to polymorphisms in GST enzymes. Several polymorphisms in genes that encode GSTs may contribute to resistance to alkylating agents. GSTT1, GSTP1 and GSTM1 show a high degree of polymorphisms, primarily, single nucleotide polymorphisms (SNPs) and less frequently, deletions [23]. Altered polymorphic frequency of genes encoding these proteins was shown to be risk factors for several cancers [16, 24].

Genetically determined deficiencies of the GST M1 or GST T1 genes were shown to as risk factors for several cancers because of their role in enzymatic detoxification of xenobiotics [23]. Two SNPs in GSTP1, the changes in codon 105 from Ile to Val, and in codon 114 from Ala to Val, affect enzyme activity. Proteins of four different alleles, GSTP1*A, GSTP1*B, GSTP1*C and GSTP1*D, are significantly different in their ability to metabolize anti-cancer drugs including alkylating agents. For example, GSTP1*A plays a role in the development of resistance to cisplatin by enhancing the capacity of the cell to form platinum–GSH conjugates. In addition, there are also evidences that the GSTP1 variants affect the response to therapy, presumably, a result of the decreased ability to metabolize/detoxify the alkylating agents used in the therapy [25]. Homozygocity for GSTP1*B has a diminished capacity to detoxify platinum based anticancer agents. This genotype is associated with a favorable outcome in the treatment of cancer patients [26]. Furthermore, the two human GSTA1 alleles, GSTA1*A and GSTA1*B result in differential expression, with lower transcriptional activation of GSTA1*B (variant) than that of GSTA1*A (common) allele. GSTA*1 catalyzes the glutathionylation of several alkylating agents, more effectively than GSTA1*B. In breast cancer patients treated with cyclophosphamide-containing combination chemotherapy, it has been shown that the patients with the homozygous GSTA1*B/1*B genotype had a better five-year survival than those with other more active GSTA1 genotypes [27].

Altered Drug Metabolism

Modified activation and inactivation of alkylating drugs are implicated in human tumor resistance. For instance, resistance to cyclophosphamide is associated with decreased conversion of this drug to its cytotoxic derivative. Certain alkylating agents such as cyclophosphamide are prodrug which must be converted to its cytotoxic forms by the targeted tumor or by other tissues. Cyclophosphamide is converted to phosphoramide mustard to act as a cytotoxic agent. Aldehyde dehydrogenase (ALDH), which is a drug metabolizing enzyme converts aldophosphamide, a metabolite of cyclophosphamide, to an acid which does not attack DNA. Thus, ALDH activity can protect cells from the cytotoxic effects of cyclophosphamide, preventing the decomposition of aldophosphamide to its cytotoxic derivative, phosphoramide mustard. Increased ALDH expression and high cytoplasmic ALDH enzyme activity were suggested as the cause of resistance to cyclophosphamid in murine, rat, human breast, colon, and ovarian tumor cells and leukemia cells [28, 29]. In vitro experiments indicated that inhibition of ALDH activity in vivo sensitizes tumors to cyclophosphamide therapy.

In addition to ALDH, several members of the CYP family such as CYP2C19 and CYP2B6 are also involved in the activation of cyclophosphamide and resistance to this drug is associated with reduced expression of these CYPs [30]. Various studies were performed to examine the relation between CYP2B6 polymorphisms and drug resistance. A correlation determined between CYP2B6 polymorphism and response to doxorubicin-cyclophosphamide therapy which is an effective treatment for early-stage breast cancer. Bray et al., [31] demonstrated that CYP2B6*2, CYP2B6*8, CYP2B6*9, and CYP2B6*4 variant alleles are associated with unresponsiveness to the treatment in breast cancer and a worse outcome.

Increased DNA Repair Capacity or Tolerance to DNA Damage

DNA repair is protective against carcinogenesis in healthy individuals however, it may play an important role in the development of resistance to chemotherapy in cancer patients. The capacity of a cancer cell to repair various types of DNA damage can determine the resistance to chemotherapeutic drugs that induce DNA damage. Enhanced activity of DNA repair capacity in tumor cells may underlie in the development of resistance to many of alkylating agents. Although response to DNA damage is a complex process involving multiple DNA repair, cell survival and cell death pathways, this response is basically either repair or cell death. Therefore, an important mechanism that helps tumor cell to avoid death induced by alkylating anticancer drugs is the activation of reparative processes in cells. Alterations in enzymes involved in DNA repair or changes in the repair capacity may allow the tumor cell to remain viable and subsequently lead to chemoresistance to alkylating drugs. Finally, the repair rate of alkylated DNA appears as an obvious mechanism of resistance to certain anti-neoplastic chemotherapeutic alkylating agents.

Numerous DNA repair pathways and their related proteins have been described to mediate the resistance to alkylating agent chemotherapy. Five main repair systems for damaged DNA are present in human cells. All of the repair systems have been described to mediate resistance to alkylating agents. Drug resistance is associated with increased DNA repair capacity. Table I shows the diversity of the mechanisms of cellular resistance to alkylating agents with respect to DNA repair.

As shown in the Table 1, there is a diversity for the mechanisms contributing to cellular resistance to alkylating agents. Resistance by enhanced MGMT repair activity has been the subject of intensive investigations. The interindividual variations in different pathways of DNA repair influence the chemosensitivity of tumor cells toward to DNA-reactive cytotoxic drugs.

Alkylating agents can transfer methyl or ethyl groups to a guanine, thereby modify the base and change its pairing specificity for cytosine during DNA replication. One of the major mechanisms used by the cell for the excision of these damaged bases is the direct repair pathway, which is typified by the DNA repair protein O^6-alkylguanine–DNA alkyltransferase (AGT, also called as O^6-methylguanine DNA methyltransferase, MGMT). This DNA repair protein encoded by MGMT gene is widely expressed in normal human tissues and it is not part of a repair complex, acts alone. This enzyme rapidly reverses alkylation at the O^6 position of guanine by removing the alkyl/ methyl group from the damaged base. It transfers the alkyl group from the O^6-guanine on DNA to an active cysteine within its own sequence in a reaction [33]. The enzyme repairs O^6-alkylguanine and O^4-alkylthymine adducts formed in DNA which is exposed to alkylating agents such as temozolomide, streptozotocin, procarbazine, dacarbazine, ethylnitrosourea, diethylnitrosamine, and nitrosoureas [34]. Several sites in DNA were described as the target for alkylation by these compounds, with the most frequent site the O^6 position of guanine. These alkylating agents can form lethal double-strand crosslinks. However, MGMT reduces the toxicity of alkylating agents by reversing the formation of adducts at the O^6 position of guanine [35]. Therefore, MGMT-mediated repair of damaged bases protects cells from the cytotoxic effects of these DNA lesions and thus causes to drug resistance in cancer cells treated with alkylating agents.

Table 1. Overview of cancer-cell-specific mechanisms of drug resistance to alkylating agents with respect to DNA repair

DNA repair pathway	Mechanism of drug resistance	Alkylating agents
1- Direct removal of DNA lesions	Enhanced O^6-methylguanine DNA methyltransferase (MGMT) activity	Bis-chloroethylnitrosourea, dacarbazine, temozolomide, and streptozotocin
2- Base excision repair	Induced X-ray cross complementation group 1 gene (XRCC1)	Chlorambucil, mitomycin C, mafosfamide, and 1,3-bis(2-chloroethyl)-1-nitrosourea
3- Nucleotide excision repair	Increased DNA damage repair by enhanced expression of ERCC1, XPC and XPF	chlorambucil and cisplatinum
4- DNA mismatch repair	The loss of function of the DNA-mismatch repair proteins MSH2 and MLH1	cisplatinum, busulfan, procarbazine, and temozolomide
5-Double strand break repair	Homologous recombination confers alkylating agent resistance.	nitrogen mustard, chlorambucil

Adapted from reference 32.

Beyond direct removal of alkyl group, the MGMT repair protein also plays a role along with MMR and BER in processing alkylation induced DNA damage. The protective effect of MGMT against alkylating agents has been demonstrated in experimental model systems [36, 37]. For example, in the study using MGMT knockout mice, primary mouse embryo fibroblasts and bone marrow cells were significantly more sensitive to toxic effects of the chemotherapeutic alkylating agents [38]. On the other hand, transgenic mice overexpressing MGMT were more resistant to alkylating agent–induced carcinogenesis [39]. In addition, introduction of human MGMT gene into enzyme-deficient cells confers potent resistance to certain alkylating agents. Several clinical studies on brain tumors suggest that there is an inverse relationship between MGMT activity and response to therapy in patients receiving some alkylating agents such as BCNU and temozolomide [40, 41].

Different pathways of DNA repair are polymorphic and vary interindividually. Accordingly, MGMT activity was found to be varied ~220-fold among individuals in cultured strains and primary samples. The interindividual variations in MGMT influence the chemosensitivity of tumor cells toward DNA-reactive cytotoxic drugs. Tumor cells can be classified into two groups depending on the relative level of MGMT. Cells with low or absent MGMT activity are quite sensitive to alkylating agents. In tumors that are more sensitive to alkylating agent-based chemotherapy, MGMT-deficient phenotype is relatively frequent and is the causative molecular abnormality in the majority of cases. Nevertheless, cells containing relatively high levels of MGMT activity are consequently resistant to alkylating agents by blunting the therapeutic effect of them [42, 43]. MGMT inhibitors such as O^6-benzylguanine allow to potentiate cytotoxic action of alkylating agents, but only in tumor cells with high levels of enzyme activity. O^6-benzylguanine is pseudo substrate and inactivator of MGMT. It reacts with MGMT by transferring the benzyl group to the active site-cysteine and causes an irreversible inactivation of the enzyme. Cellular MGMT can be depleted by this way. O^6-benzylguanine is not toxic alone at therapeutic levels, but efficiently renders the tumor cells 2- to 14-fold more sensitive to alkylating agents. This establishes the potential therapeutic effect of O^6-benzylguanine as an enhancer of these drugs.

In the course of tumor development, gene silencing by DNA methylation is an early and important mechanism. Cancer arises because of inactivation of tumor-suppressor genes by promoter hypermethylation. In human cancer, loss of MGMT function is most frequently caused by promoter methylation of the MGMT gene rather than its inactivation via mutation [44, 45]. Hypermethylation of CpG islands in the MGMT promoter prevents binding of transcription factor and subsequent gene expression, and lowers cellular ability to repair of damaged DNA in tumor cells. Epigenetic silencing of this gene has been reported in a variety of cancers, including glioblastomas, colon cancer, gastric carcinoma, non-small cell lung cancer, head and neck squamous cell carcinoma as well as many other cancer types [46-49]. Tumor cells with unmethylated MGMT promoters are more resistant to alkylating agents, while tumor cells with hypermethylated MGMT promoters are more sensitive to alkylating agents. From a clinical standpoint, Monika et al. [50] reported that patients with high-grade gliomas with methylated MGMT promoters have a better survival when treated with temozolomide. An increasing number of studies provide evidences linking promoter methylation of MGMT to loss of protein expression with respect to alkylating agents, in particular, temozolomide. Some authors suggest that MGMT promoter methylation status might have predictive value for clinical response to alkylating chemotherapy [51, 52]. MGMT-currently is used as a predictor of successful alkylation chemotherapy for various tumor, especially for glioblastoma.

Another mechanism of resistance to alkylating agents is the base excision repair (BER) pathway which typically repairs oxidized and alkylated nucleobases. Alkylation adducts such as N^7-methylguanine and N^3-methyladenine are the targets of this repair mechanism. PolyADP–ribose polymerase (PARP) is involved in this process. X-ray cross complementation group 1 (XRCC1) interacts with DNA ligase III and forms complexes with DNA polymerase B and PARP to participate in the base excision repair pathway. PARP-1 proteins interact with DNA single-strand breaks and have a particular role nucleotide repair pathway as well as the base excision repair pathway. Poly (ADP-ribose) polymerase (PARP-1) which is the founding member of the PARP family catalyzes the polymerization of ADP-ribose units from donor NAD^+ molecules on target proteins. Enzymatic activity of PARP-1 is stimulated by some undamaged DNA structures, nucleosomes, and a variety of protein-binding partners as well as damaged DNA, and poly(ADP-ribosyl)ation may alter the activity of acceptor protein [53, 54]. In general, in response to DNA damage generated either exogenously or endogenously, PARP-1 interacts physically and functionally with various proteins involved in multiple DNA repair pathways and may act to recruit repair proteins to sites of DNA damage (e.g., XRCC1 in BER, DNA-dependent protein kinase in double strand break repair) [55]. As might be expected, tumor cells with normal BER pathway and PARP-1 activity rapidly repair DNA adducts induced by alkylating agents. It was shown that PARP-1 knockout animals are sensitive to alkylating agents [56].

Among DNA repair pathways, nucleotide excision repair (NER) is a versatile repair pathway involved in the removal of a variety of bulky DNA lesions. NER pathways recognize and remove damaged nucleotide segments from a single strand and then resynthesize the new DNA segment. Components of the NER complex also play a role in the repair of double strand breaks. Platinum agents such as oxaliplatin and cisplatin form bulky DNA adducts in cells and the damage are predominantly removed by this repair pathway. Mammalian cells that have defects in the NER system are hypersensitive to alkylating agents. A study of various alkylating agent-resistance models was shown enhanced DNA adduct repair capacity with respect to NER complex [57]. Evidences from several laboratories indicated that one of the causes of resistance to alkylating agent-based chemotherapies may include alterations of expression levels in several components of NER protein complex [58]. Although approximately 30 proteins participate to NER process, it is known that the excision repair cross-complementing 1 (ERCC1) protein has a crucial role in the incision process and is an important rate-limiting factor [59]. In vitro studies showed that ERCC1 mRNA expression is elevated in oxaliplatin-resistant colorectal and ovarian carcinoma cell lines [60, 61]. Data from experimental cell models were shown that suppression of ERCC1 expression by using antisense ERCC1 RNA enhances or restores platinum sensitivity [57]. Some clinical trials in ovarian, gastric and non-small-cell lung carcinoma reported that increased levels of ERCC1 correlated with poor response to platinum-based chemotherapy [62, 63]. In addition, it has been demonstrated that the aberrant CpG island methylation in ERCC1 promoter region exists in human glioma cell lines as well as clinical glioma samples and it is associated with cisplatin chemosensitivity [64]. Nowadays, ERCC1 stands out as a potential predictive marker for cisplatin-based chemotherapy. On the other hand, overexpression of xeroderma pigmentosum group A (XPA) which is another central component of NER complex was found to be associated with increased resistance to cisplatin [62]. A study carried out by Wu et al. [65] reported that transfection with antisense XPA RNA of human lung adenocarcinoma cells can decrease the XPA mRNA level and sensitize tumor cells to cisplatin. They suggested that enhanced sensitivity can be attributed to the reduced NER capacity.

DNA mismatch repair system (MMR) is responsible for recognition and correction of erroneous DNA base pairing during DNA replication.

Inactivation of MMR greatly increases spontaneous mutation rates. An additional role of MMR pathway is to trigger cell cycle arrest and apoptosis, if repair is unsuccessful. Several proteins (hMLH1, hPMS2, hMSH2, hMSH2 and hMSH6) are included in this pathway. The MMR proteins are critical for the maintenance of genomic stability by excising single-base mismatches and insertion-deletion loops on newly synthesized DNA [66].

The MMR system plays a significant role in the repair of DNA damage induced by various classes of clinically (or experimentally) active alkylating drugs including monofunctional alkylators such as temozolomide, dacarbazine, N-methyl-N'-nitro-N-nitrosoguandine (an experimental drug); bifunctional alkylators such as the platinum analogues, cisplatin and carboplatin [67]. Cytotoxicity of O^6-methyl guanine created by alkylating agents is also mediated by MMR pathway. During DNA replication, DNA polymerase mispairs O^6-methylguanine with thymine, creating a distortion in the DNA double helix. Then, components of MMR complex recognize and repair the mispaired thymine. If O^6-methylguanine remains in place, MMR system may lead to the induction of double-strand breaks and apoptosis. Mammalian cells with an effective defense system are nearly 100-fold more sensitive to alkylating agents as compared to their MMR-deficient counterparts [68]. MMR-deficient cells are nearly 100 times more resistant to killing by alkylating agents. Therefore, the MMR system plays a key role in the killing the cell in response to alkylating agents. Defects in the MMR system were associated with resistance to alkylating agents, possibly by the development of inability to recognize the mismatching of O^6-methylguanine to thymine and to initiate the cycle of futile repair attempts, cell-cycle arrest and apoptosis. Defects in MMR may be either inherited, as in the case of hereditary nonpolyposis colorectal carcinoma, which is caused by mutations in hMLH or hMSH2 genes, or may occur through epigenetic silencing of an essential MMR gene [58]. In experimental cell models, colon cancer cells are resistant to alkylating agents like as to other cell lines deficient in hMLH1. Resistance to alkylating agents associated with epigenetic silencing of MMR genes seems to occur most often through hMLH1 promoter hypermethylation in CpG islands, as described in different types of cancers [69]. MLH1 expression is not only increased by DNA damage but also seems to be linked to apoptotic pathways. Cell lines with deficient hMLH1 via promoter methylation were shown to be resistant to the cytotoxic effects of alkylating agents such as temozolomide, dacarbazine and cisplatin. Furthermore, it has been also been reported that *MSH6* mutations were frequent in recurrent glioblastomas that have been treated with alkylating agents [70] .

Another mechanism found to contribute to increased DNA repair capacity is mediated by increased activity of topoisomerase II. The alterations of topoisomerase II activity were also described to be associated with resistance to alkylating agents [71]. Mammalian DNA topoisomerases are nuclear enzymes that regulate topological changes in DNA and that is essential for transcription, replication and chromosome segregation during the cell division. The level of this enzyme is high in proliferating cells, and very low in quiescent cells. In certain studies, a correlation was observed between high expression of topoisomerase II and resistance to certain DNA-damaging agents [72, 73]. It was proposed that DNA cross-links in resistant cells to alkylating agents could increase the affinity of topoisomerase II and induce the topological change in the DNA template [73]. Thus this enzyme may play a role in resistance to alkylators by facilitating DNA repair.

In addition to the factors discussed above, several different resistance factors may also contribute to increased DNA repair. Data obtained from studies using cell lines and patient samples with acquired resistance to alkylating agents suggested that resistance to certain alkylating agents are associated with overexpression of the DNA damage recognition protein HMG1 and of damaged-DNA-binding-protein-2 (DDB2) [2].

Impairment/Deficiency of Cellular Mechanisms Causing Cytotoxicity of Alkylating Agent-Mediated DNA Damage

Reduced Apoptotic Response and Alkylating Agent Resistance

The DNA-damaging events caused by alkylating agents initiate apoptosis which is required for antineoplastic activity. Therefore, increase of DNA damage tolerance, and failure of cell death pathways may contribute to the development of human tumor resistance. Toleranced phenotype to DNA damage induced by alkylating agents may be a consequence of decreased expression or inactivation of one or more components of the programmed cell death pathway.

Apoptosis, or programmed cell death, is a major control mechanism and a natural barrier to cancer development by which cells die if DNA damage is not repaired. Resistance to apoptosis or evasion of apoptosis is closely linked to tumorigenesis. Therefore, induction of apoptosis in tumor cells is one of the major goals of current anti-cancer treatments. Cells exposed to cytotoxic levels of DNA damaging agents exhibit some typical characteristics of apoptosis such as chromatin condensation, shrinkage of the cells and nuclear fragmentation. Although the most alkylating agents are very potent inducers of apoptosis, resistance may develop. Resistance is implied when tumor cells fail to undergo apoptosis at clinically relevant drug concentrations. There is a critical balance between cell cycle arrest and cell death following chemotherapy. Apoptotic deregulation may lead to chemoresistance and survival of cancer cells despite the successfully targeted anti-cancer drugs. There is accumulating evidence for the concept that tumour resistance to alkylating agent may be mediated by enhanced tolerance to DNA damage via impaired apoptotic response. Resistance to induction of apoptosis by alkylating agents can be acquired through chronic drug exposure or it can occur itself as an intrinsic phenomenon [74].

Understanding the regulation of apoptosis will help us to better evaluate its impact on development of resistance to alkylating agent. Apoptosis is a tightly regulated form of cell death, which can be triggered by two different types of signals or two main pathways: intracellular stress signals and extracellular ligands [75]. Both the extrinsic, with another word receptor-mediated pathway, and the intrinsic (called as mitochondrial pathway) of apoptosis are regulated by the tumor suppressor p53 (also known as protein 53). The extrinsic pathway can be initiated by the activation of cell surface death receptors following binding of extracellular ligands such as members of the tumor necrosis factor (TNF) family. The mitochondrial intrinsic pathway is activated by stress signals such as DNA damage, hypoxia or loss of survival signals. Bcl-2 (B-cell CLL/Lymphoma 2) family proteins mediate the mitochondrial regulation of apoptosis by promoting or inhibiting permeabilization of mitochondrial outer membrane, and consequently release of proapoptotic mitochondrial factors. Function of the pro-apoptotic proteins (Bax, Bak, Bok, Bid, Bad, Bim, Bik, Blk, Hrk, Noxa, and Puma) which are the key regulators of the apoptosis-mediating mitochondrial cytochrome c release is regulated by antiapoptotic Bcl-2 proteins such as Bcl-2, Bcl-XL, and Mcl-1. These proteins act in the form of homodimers (such as Bcl-2/Bcl-2) or heterodimers (e.g. Bcl-2/Bax), either in an antiapoptotic or proapoptotic manner, and may regulate outer mitochondrial membrane integrity and function. The ratio of anti- to pro-apoptotic molecules determines the cellular susceptibility to death signals by titrating one another's function. Only an excess level of homodimers can either inhibit (e.g. Bcl-2/Bcl-2) or induce (e.g. Bax/Bax) apoptosis.

Dysfunction of mitochondria induced by DNA damage and other genotoxic factors may lead to permeability of mitochondrial outer membrane that results the release of caspase-activating molecules. Caspases is a family of cysteine proteases that cleave after aspartic acid residues. They are also involved in the extrinsic pathway. Caspases categorized as initiator which cleave other caspases lead to cell death by catalyzing proteolysis. In this sequential process, the alterations disrupting the normal apoptotic response to alkylating agent-mediated DNA damage may result in chemoresistance due to impaired apoptosis.

The critical roles of loss of normal p53 function, up-regulation of Bcl-2 or Bcl-XL, or overexpression of epidermal growth factor receptor (EGFR) in alkylating agent resistance were elucidated by numerous in vitro studies [53, 76]. P53 is a crucial element involved in the regulation of cell cycle arrest and cell death. P53 tumor suppressor protein acts as a critical damage sensor. Although tumors acquire resistance to apoptosis through several strategies, mutational loss-of p53 function results in elimination of this damage sensor from the apoptosis-inducing system, and this is frequently observed in tumor cells. P53 gene is mutated in approximately 50% of human cancers. Mutated p53 gene is often associated with advanced tumor grade and poor prognosis in many forms of cancer. P53 facilitates DNA repair before DNA replication and it is also known as an important determinant of the pathway which triggers the apoptosis as a response to DNA damage. Although apoptosis may occur either p53-dependent or independent, frequently the cellular response to DNA damage is regulated by p53 [44]. Ectopic expression of wild type p53 leads to induction of rapid apoptosis or irreversible growth arrest in many tumor cell lines [77]. It is believed that reintroduction of wild p53 into p53 mutant tumor cells can make the tumor more sensitive to treatment through the induction of apoptosis [78]. Therefore, drugs which induce DNA damage, would lead to p53-mediated cell death. On the other hand, several experiments were reported that inability of p53 in the induction of apoptosis in cells contributes to drug resistance, allowing cells to replicate with damaged DNA [79]. In the same way, several studies suggest that intrinsic or acquired resistance to classical alkylating agents and platinum-based drugs can be attributed at least in part to altered expression and/or mutation of p53.

However, conflicting results were also reported for the role of mutant p53 in determination of the chemosensitivity. Although the specific contribution of p53 to clinical resistance is still uncertain, emerging evidences suggest that loss of p53 function is strongly associated with clinically resistant and aggressive tumors [80]. This may be more significant cause of chemoresistance to alkylating drugs observed in the clinically as compared to other drug-specific mechanisms.

As respect with the fact that attenuation of apoptosis may affect cellular sensitivity to DNA damaging agents in cells, down regulation of Bcl-2 family proteins contributes not only to disease pathogenesis but also to the development of resistance to cytotoxic therapies in human cancers. Because apoptotic signaling is a result of the homeostasis of the Bcl-2 proteins, and modifications of these family members would influence the response of tumor cells to chemotherapeutic treatment. Analysis of gene expression profiles following exposure to some alkylating agents revealed that overexpression of Bcl-2 or Bcl-XL may prevent loss of the mitochondrial transmembrane potential and prolong cell survival in some tumor cells. Dysfunction of the pro-apoptotic Bcl-2 members can contribute to alkylating drug resistance. In addition, impairment in the protease effectors' phase of apoptosis may also lead to chemo- resistance to alkylating agents. In this case, caspases are involved in the development of drug resistance. It was reported that cisplatin resistance in ovarian cancer cell lines is associated with the overexpression of anti-apoptotic protein Bcl-2 and down regulation of caspase-3 activity [81]. In another study, a splice variant form of caspase-3 was found to be overexpressed in chemoresistant breast carcinomas, and is particularly associated with poor response to neoadjuvant cyclophosphamide-containing treatment cyclophosphamide [82]. Although overexpression of Bcl-2 and/or Bcl-XL was found to be correlated with poor clinical outcome in various different solid tumor types as well as in hematological malignancies, it should be noted that the contributory role of proteins of the Bcl-2 family in chemoresistance to alkylating drug was mainly obtained from *in vitro* models using cancer derived cell lines. Therefore, clinical relevance of apoptosis resistance observed in model systems should be confirmed in future studies.

Non-Apoptotic Deaths and Alkylating Agent Resistance

Apoptosis is not the unique mechanism in the killing of tumor cells by anti-cancer therapy. Tumor killing is achieved by further mechanisms such as autophagy, mitotic catastrophe and necrosis. A number of alkylating agents were observed to induce acute necrotic tumour cell death and autophagy in human cancer cell lines. Several studies have shown that modulation of autophagy sensitizes lymphoma and brain tumor cells to alkylating agent therapy [83, 84].

Autophagy, as in apoptosis, is crucial for cellular homeostasis, normally operates at low basal levels in cells and can be strongly induced in certain stresses such as various infectious diseases, neurodegeneration, metabolic stresses and cancer. Autophagy is a catabolic process characterized by the formation of autophagic vesicles that segregate damaged organelles and proteins and target them for degradation through fusion with the lysosomes. The bulk degradation of cellular material through autophagy allows cells to recycle the nutrients required for energy production during starvation and stress [85]. Autophagy is regulated by a limited number of highly conserved genes called ATGs (for AuTophaGy gene). On the other hand, an excessive level of autophagy is proposed to promote cell death due to the over-consumption of critical cellular constituents such as poly(ADP-ribose) polymerase (PARP) and ATP.

Autophagy is believed to have an important role in tumorigenesis. In vivo experiments in established in animals showed that autophagy has a tumor suppressive role in the early stages of tumorigenesis [83]. At this stage, the rate of protein synthesis in cancer cells is significantly higher than protein degradation to maintain the tumor growth. Furthermore, it is thought that autophagy decreases the mutation rate and suppresses oncogenesis by eliminating damaged organelles that produce genotoxic stresses such as free radicals. At the early stages of tumor development, induction of autophagy in cell reduces tumorigenic capacity by expression of beclin 1 (BECN1), a mammalian orthologue of the yeast autophagy-related gene Atg6. It was shown that introduction of BECN1 into MCF7 breast cancer cells induced autophagy and inhibited tumorigenicity [86]. Although autophagy is suppressed during the early stages of tumorigenesis, it is proposed to play a tumor-promoting role during the later stages of tumor growth. Autophagy is believed to be necessary for the survival of cancer cells so that its induction allows cancer cells that are located in the central areas of the tumour to survive in low-nutrient and low oxygen conditions which load the stress to tumor cells. Thus, it is increasingly appreciated that autophagy provides a selective advantage to tumor cell to cope with stress.

A number of clinically available cancer therapeutics including DNA damaging chemotherapy are based on induction of autophagy in cancer cells derived from tissues such as breast, colon, prostate and brain. Temozolomide induces autophagy, but not apoptosis, in vivo in glioblastoma models [87]. On the other hand, autophagy plays an important role in determining the response of tumor cells to therapy. There is an evidence that autophagy in response to alkylating drug therapy can contribute to the tumor cell's ability to resist apoptosis. In this study, inhibition of autophagy improved the response of tumors to alkylating agents [83]. In addition, a few studies showed that autophagy-related proteins such as Beclin-1, Atg5 and LC3 were low in resistant cells following temozomolide treatment, and temozolomide-induced autophagy might contribute to the development of resistance [84]. Furthermore, in another study, it was found that the autophagic index (mean number of autophagic vesicles per cell) is high in tumor biopsies obtained from metastatic melanoma patients [88]. The findings indicate that increased autophagy is associated with poor prognosis and resistance to temozolomide in patients with advanced melanoma. However, there is no clear agreement on whether therapy-induced autophagy contributes to tumor cell death or represents a mechanism of resistance to alkylating agent-mediated cell death.

Newer Molecular Mechanisms Linked to Alkylating Agent Resistance

Tumor Microenvironment in Alkylating Agent Resistance

The limitations of clinical chemotherapy including alkylating agents are ascribed primarily to mechanisms that mediate drug resistance at the cellular level. However, an increasing number of reports are suggested that mechanisms involving tumor microenvironment may also mediate resistance of solid tumors and hematologic malignancies to chemotherapy. Some authors now claim that tumor resistance is not only a process involving epigenetic or genetic events, but also depends on the microenvironment. The tumor microenvironment is comprised of normal stromal cells and non-cellular components including extracellular matrix (ECM) and soluble factors such as cytokines and growth factors. Communication between cells in both normal and tumor microenvironment is essential for cell growth. The tumor microenvironment is characterized by acidity, regions of hypoxia and gradients in the rate of cell proliferation. Tumor cells as well as normal cells are influenced by the extrinsic factors provided by the microenvironment itself through intercellular communication via direct contact. Interaction between cells (tumor-tumor cell, tumor-stromal cell and tumor-ECM) contributes to tumor cell survival mediated by this contact. Besides this, soluble factors such as cytokines and growth factors in the tumor microenvironment provide further signals for tumorigenesis. Moreover, the interaction between microenvironmental components and tumor cells can also influence the survival of cancer cells during treatment that can contribute to development of drug resistance. All of these environmental factors can influence the tumor cell sensitivity to drug treatment [89]. Recently, there is increasing interest for possible role of tumor microenvironment for drug resistance. Therefore, the role of tumor microenvironment in the development of resistance to anti-neoplastic chemotherapeutic alkylating agents is discussed briefly below.

Hypoxia and Alkylating Agent Resistance

The oxygenation level within a tumor is not homogeneous, and poorly oxygenated and hypoxic regions are substantially increased in most solid tumors compared to normal tissue. As result of the limited vasculature of tumors, in the distant regions from blood vessels at which hypoxia occurs, the oxygen concentration may fall to zero. The resultant hypoxia increases the mutation rate and the expression of hundreds of genes in tumor cells. This leads to activation of genes which are associated with angiogenesis and cell survival resulting in the selection of mutations that make cells more resistant to apoptosis and less responsive to cancer therapy. Therefore, up or down regulation of various genes induced by hypoxia may result in the expansion of populations of cells with altered biochemical pathways which may be involved in resistance to alkylating chemotherapeutic agents. For example, hypoxia is known to down regulate expression of the anti-apoptotic protein BCL-2 in some chemotherapy-resistant human cell lines.

pH and Alkylating Agent Resistance

The pH in the tumor microenvironment can influence the cytotoxicity of anticancer drugs. In addition, factors such as diet, other medications, as well as certain medical conditions that affect pH may impact drug efficacy. The extracellular pH in tumors is often low than normal tissues and the intracellular pH of tumor cells is neutral to alkaline. Alterations in acidity of extracellular or intracellular environment of tumor cells can enhance the uptake and cytotoxicity of some chemotherapeutic agents. For example, weakly acidic alkylating agents such as chlorambucil or cyclophosphamide are more concentrated in the relatively neutral intracellular space. Tumor extracellular pH is increased by bicarbonate and lowered by glucose administration. For instance, cisplatin uptake is markedly increased at low extracellular pH. Meanwhile, it is known that some agents such as mannitol and NaCl which are used to decrease cisplatin nephrotoxicity, decrease cisplatin uptake and cytotoxicity.

Besides these, binding of drug to proteins in blood can also contribute to resistance. Protein-bound platinum is much less cytotoxic than free cisplatin. The tumor cells can influence the associated stroma and other surrounding cells by altered expression of surface receptors or release of secretory factors, which can lead to formation of a tumor-specific extracellular matrix. Therefore, the extracellular matrix is altered during tumor progression. Components in the extracellular matrix of tumor may also vary from one location to another in the same tumor. The distribution of many drugs within tumors may vary depending on the local milieu of the cancer cells. The three-dimensional structure of tissue itself depending on the differences in amount and composition of extracellular matrix may modify the responsiveness of tumors to exogenous apoptotic stimuli. In this regard, it can also influence the sensitivity of constituent cells to chemotherapy. For example, tumor cells grown in contact with each other are more resistant to alkylating agents than the same cells after disaggregation [90]. Teicher et al. [90] showed that mammary tumors made resistant to alkylating agents in vivo were sensitized to cytotoxic drugs once removed from the animal. In addition, it is generally believed that ECM proteins such as various collagens and laminins, which are elevated in tumor microenvironment can protect cancer cells from chemotherapeutic drugs-induced apoptosis. Adhesion to these ECM components in the tumor microenvironment was shown to prevent various drug-induced apoptosis [91].

Cellular Adhesion and Alkylating Agent Resistance

Although anchorage-independency for growth and survival is considered an essential feature of malignant cells, adhesive interactions between same cell types were shown to may confer resistance to alkylating agents. This phenomenon, known as cell adhesion–mediated drug resistance, is observed in a variety of cancer types [77]. Several experiments suggest the integrins as being closely involved in resistance to alkylating agent chemotherapy [91]. Resistance-promoting effects by integrin-mediated adhesion to ECM are observed in various cancers, including pancreas, ovary, prostate, breast, liver, brain and leukemia [92]. The majority of integrins bind to extracellular matrix proteins such as fibronectin that is the ligand for at least 10 integrin molecules. Interaction of integrin with fibronectin can also elicit signaling responses in cancer cells, affecting their behavior. Experimental findings indicate the contributory roles of β1 integrins and fibronectin in apoptotic suppression and cell survival. Recent studies have shown the importance of these adhesion molecules (integrins and cadherins) in drug resistance development [93, 94]. Integrin-specific adhesion of cells to fibronectin are shown to confer resistance to alkylating agents via alterations in cyclin dependent kinase inhibitors such as p27kip1 [95]. In addition, an increased expression and/or high affinity state of α4β1 (and/or α5β1) integrin and fibronectin adhesion were reported to be associated with tolerance of cancer cells to various chemotherapeutic drugs including certain alkylating agents [96]. Hazlehurst et al. [97] also revealed that β1-integrin adhesion to fibronectin protects myeloma cells from melphalan-induced apoptosis by protecting mitochondria from drug-induced DNA damage. It was shown that β 1-integrin-mediated adhesion could modulate cellular localization and availability of several apoptotic regulators (such as CASP8, c-FLIPL and BIM), protecting tumor cells from apoptosis [77].

The interaction between the tumor microenvironment and tumor cells also confers drug resistance by soluble factor such as cytokines and growth factors produced in the microenvironment as well as by direct contact. Many soluble factors act as a survival factor in both solid tumors and hematologic malignancies. They may confer drug resistance by stimulating cell survival and growth. For example, interleukin (IL)-6, a cytokine secreted by bone marrow stromal cells, activates multiple cell signalling pathways that promote myeloma cell proliferation, survival and resistance to chemotherapy. Activation of Stat3 pathway by IL-6 confers protection from Fas-mediated apoptosis by up-regulating the antiapoptotic protein Bcl-XL. It was shown that IL-6 confers resistance to prostate carcinoma cells against cisplatin cytotoxicity [98]. In addition, it was reported that inhibition of IL-6 by the anti-IL-6 monoclonal antibody in combination with standard or high dose melphalan may improve clinical outcomes [99]. On the other hand, findings of the experiments in which cell survival pathways initiated by soluble factors are inhibited with various inhibitors revealed the appearance of drug resistant phenotype, and this might be derived from existence of other drug resistant mechanisms.

Cancer Stem Cells in Alkylating Agents Resistance

During recent years, an increasing number of reports have suggested that a tumor mass includes not only dividing tumor cell clones, but also tumor-initiating cells referred as cancer stem cells (CSCs). These are rare tumor cells (approximately 1%). These minor tumor cell populations with stem cell properties are capable of maintaining continuous tumor growth and may have an essential role in tumour formation and maintenance. A consensus panel convened by the American Association of Cancer Research defined a CSC as a cell within a tumor that possesses the capacity to self-renew and to cause the heterogeneous lineages of cancer cells that comprise the tumor [100] . Although there are many controversies related to the cancer stem cell paradigm, there are also increasing evidences for the existence of CSCs in both haematopoietic and solid cancers such as breast, brain, lung, and colon cancer as well as commercial cell lines. Besides this, there are experimental evidences to support relevance of the CSC in drug resistance [101-104]. Investigations in various cancers such as glioblastoma and breast cancer support the idea that cancer stem cells are more resistant to chemotherapy as compared to rapidly proliferating progenitor cells and differentiated tumor cells. Additionally, the CSC model also provides an improved understanding of tumor resistance to alkylating agents [15].

Recently, a set of papers suggest that cancer stem cells may contribute to certain anti-neoplastic chemotherapeutic alkylating agents. Accumulating evidence suggests that several emerging concepts might be important in the drug-resistant phenotype of various cell types. Cancer stem cells from brain tumors that express the neural stem cell surface marker CD133+ were found to be more resistant to temozolomide and 1,3-bis(2-chloroethyl)-1-nitrosourea (BCNU) as compared to their non-cancer SC counterparts (CD133−)[23]. Furthermore, CD133 expression in recurrent glioblastomas tissue obtained from five patients was higher than those in a newly diagnosed patients, suggesting the CD133+ cancer SCs were better able to survive [23]. There are multiple reports that cancer stem cells express high levels of MGMT, known to be involved in alkylating agent resistance.

In general, cancer cells produce increased amounts of reactive oxygen species (ROS) because of the altered metabolic demand, so they are more vulnerable to further oxidative stress produced by exogenous ROS-generating agents such as TMZ. It is known that TMZ-resistant tumor cells under conditions of oxidative stress generate substantially less ROS, reduce states 2 and 4 of mitochondrial respiration [45]. On the other hand, both CSC induced ROS-adaptive response and tumor cell response may also play a critical role in protection of cells against the damaging and cytotoxic effects of anticancer agents. It has been shown that breast cancer stem cells contain lower ROS levels and enhanced ROS-scavenging systems as compared with their normal counterparts [105]. Therefore, adaptive responses of cancer cells and CSCs to ROS-generating alkylating agents may be relevant in maintaining homeostasis of intracellular medium and microenvironment of tumor and in favoring cell survival.

Although chemotherapy kills most cells in a tumour, it is believed to leave cancer stem cells behind, which might be an important mechanism of resistance. How do tumour stem cells escape therapy-associated cell death? Recent studies about therapy resistance of CSC proposed distinct cellular mechanisms that may actively resist the cytotoxic effects of alkylating agents. Most chemotherapeutic drugs including DNA damaging agents target rapidly dividing tumor cells within the tumor bulk. According to a recent hypothesis, CSCs exhibit a lower rate of proliferation and therefore are not targeted by those therapeutic agents [106]. As regarding alkylating agents, anticancer treatment that targets actively proliferating cells, are less effective in killing tumour stem cells than mature 'differentiated' cancer cells. Thus, cancer stem cells may remain largely unaffected and can maintain continuous tumour growth. Other possible explanation for why cancer stem cells escape therapy-associated cell death is that they have differences in the functionality of cell cycle checkpoints and enhanced repair of drug-induced damage than non-CSCs. The mechanisms involved in drug resistance phenotype of CSCs are not completely understood, although available literature data suggest that these cells are neither resistant nor susceptible to chemotherapy per se. It is also not clear whether molecular mechanisms responsible for CSC-mediated therapeutic resistance are shared across different tumor types.

Above all, the present studies suggest that drug resistance of CSCs results from changes in different intracellular pathways, several mechanisms may be involved in this phenomenon and resistance of tumor and tumor-derived CSC against alkylating agents is much more complex than expected.

Involvement of miRNA in Resistance to Alkylating Agent

MicroRNAs (miRNAs), a class of endogenous non-protein-coding RNAs, function as important regulatory molecules in negatively regulation of gene expression. They have regulatory roles in a broad range of biological processes, including embryogenesis, differentiation, proliferation and apoptosis. Micro-RNAs influence nearly all aspects of health and diseases. miRNAs were demonstrated to play a role in the development and progression of various tumours. Several studies showed that expression profiling of miRNAs in diverse hematologic and solid tumours is altered by up-regulation or down-regulation [89, 107, 108]. The deregulation in expression profiling of miRNAs in malignant tumour cells can be caused by three main mechanisms: location of miRNAs at cancer associated genomic regions /at fragile sites, epigenetic regulation of miRNA genes, and abnormalities in miRNA processing genes and proteins [109]. The function of miRNAs in the different cancer cells can be also affected by miRNA mutations/polymorphisms. Recent evidences indicate that miRNAs can also influence tumour cell response to anticancer treatments, including alkylating agents. A strong correlation between the expression patterns of miRNAs and the potency patterns of anticancer compounds was shown [107, 108].

Up- and/or down-regulation of miRNAs may influence the expression of multiple proteins by changing expression of multiple target mRNAs, leading to variations in the chemosensitivity of cancer cells via various cellular processes. miRNAs that undergo aberrant regulation during tumorigenesis frequently alter response to chemotherapy by modulation of survival pathways and/or apoptotic response [110]. As less frequently, some miRNAs may affect other mechanisms such as drug metabolism via targeting drug transporters and drug metabolizing enzymes. Furthermore, miRNA-mediated modulation of drug targeting and DNA repair may contribute to drug resistance for alkylating agents in tumor cells. Several miRNAs are known to be associated with chemotherapeutic efficacy. One of them is miR-21, which was identified as an anti-apoptotic factor. It was found to have multiple roles in resistance to several anticancer agents. Regarding alkylating agents, a recent in vitro study demonstrated that over-expression of miR-21 protects the glioblastoma cell line against temozolomide-induced apoptosis by down-regulation of pro-apoptotic Bax, up-regulation of anti-apoptotic Bcl-2, and by a decrease in caspase-3 activity [111]. In addition, Ujifuku et al. [112] suggest that miR-195, miR-455-3p and miR-10a* may play a role in acquired temozolomide resistance in glioblastoma multiforme.

Another miRNA involved in resistance to alkylating agents is the miR-200 family which is highly expressed in endometrial and esophageal cancers. Its overexpression is correlated with cisplatin resistance [113]. In consistent with this finding, overexpression of miR-200c was found to be correlated with poor response to cisplatin-based chemotherapy in patients with esophageal cancer [114]. This study showed that miR-200c–induced resistance is mediated through the Akt pathway. More recently, a study on three microRNAs (mir-21, let-7i, and mir-16) previously implicated in cancer, demonstrated that the change in cellular levels of these miRNAs affected the potencies of a number of anticancer agents up to 4-fold depending on the compound class and cancer type [115]. Different studies revealed that miRNAs can have opposite effects towards the same anticancer agent in different tumour types, and that they can alter the efficiency of various anticancer agents differently in the same cancer cell.

On the other hand, several groups noted that there is a strong association between miR-polymorphisms and drug response. A single miR-polymorphism may contribute to the resistance of tumor cells to antitumor agents by affecting the expression of multiple genes involved in pathways regulating drug absorption, distribution, metabolism, and excretion. With regard to cisplatin, in a key experiment in which the endometrial cancer cell line HEC-1A used, Wu et al., [116] showed that a miR-200b/200c/429-binding site polymorphism in the 3' untranslated region of the AP-2α gene was associated with drug resistance.

Transcription factor AP-2 α functions as a tumor suppressor by regulating the transcription of various genes that are involved in cell proliferation and apoptosis. Cisplatin induces post-transcriptionally endogenous AP-2 α, which contributes to chemosensitivity by enhancing therapy-induced apoptosis. Enhanced expression of AP-2 α in cancer cells is known to increase the sensitivity to cisplatin. The reported findings suggest that miR-200b/miR-200c/miR-429 overexpression induces cisplatin resistance by repressing AP-2α expression in the endometrial cancer cell line HEC-1A.

Briefly, given that a single miRNA can target hundreds of mRNAs, it seems that the relationship between function of miRNAs and drug resistance is highly complex.

Other Molecules Contributing the Resistance to Alkylating Agents

The development of genomic and proteomic technologies allows us to visualize the expression of potentially all genes that may be involved in regulation of tumour cell response to chemotherapy and alkylating agent. In comparative proteomics studies, alkylating sensitive versus–resistant lines differentially expressed several proteins of interest associated with signal transduction (e.g., IP3R1, SRPK1, SAPK/JNK, Protein phosphatases 2A and 4, Hyaluronan-CD44), molecular chaperones (e.g., HSP70, HSP90-β glucose-regulated-stress-protein-78 (GRP78), protein disulfide isomerases (PDIA1, PDIA3, PDIA4, PDIA6), calnexin, heat shock protein beta-11), apoptosis inhibitors (e.g., surviving, Xiap (X-linked inhibitor of apoptosis protein) , Fas associated death domain-like interleukin-1beta-converting enzyme-like inhibitory protein (FLIP)) mitochondria (e.g., Mitochondrial-uncoupling protein-2), transcription factors (e.g., Y-box-binding protein-1 (YB-1), CCAAT-binding-transcription-factor-2 (CTF2), activating-transcription-factor-4 (ATF4), zincfinger-factor-143 (ZNF143), mitochondrial-transcription factor-A (mtTFA), Ets-1 and AP-2), cell-cycle related factors (e.g., S-phase-kinase-associated-protein-2 (SKP2), Cyclin D1) and the cell cycle checkpoint (e.g., Checkpoint-kinase-2 (Chk2)) [117].

As shown in the Table 2, overexpression of some proteins and decreased levels of others are frequently associated with alkylating agent resistance. Although there are several clinical data supporting the role of components of these pathways in alkylating agent resistance, it is still unknown which of these numerous resistance mechanisms are the most important clinically.

Conclusion

Alkylating agents are the most frequently used agents among the chemotherapics. Despite significant advances in the treatment of cancer, resistance to alkylating agents as well as various chemotherapeutics is a major handicap of the successful treatment. In this chapter, rather than the strategies for overcoming resistance, some of the mechanisms thought to be associated with resistance to alkylating agent therapy that represents multidimensional and multifactorial problem is reviewed.

Table 2. Differently expressed several proteins in alkylating agent resistant cell lines

Protein	Biological pathway	Resistance mechanism	Change (↑↓)
IP3R1, SRPK1	Signal transduction	Altered cell signaling pathways	↓
SAPK/JNK, Protein phosphatases 2A and 4, Hyaluronan-CD44,	Signal transduction	Altered cell signaling pathways	↑
DJ-1, YB-1	Transcription factor	Increased cellular survival	↑
Glutathione transferase kappa 1	Redox homeostasis and stress response	Increased drug detoxification	↑
HSP70, HSP90-β, PDIA1, PDIA3, PDIA4, PDIA6, calnexin	Stress proteins and chaperones	Increased chaperones	↑
Heat shock protein beta-11	Stress proteins and cell adhesion		↓
Rad23A, Rad51, Ribonucleotide reductase M1	DNA repair	Increased DNA damage repair	↑
Mitochondrial-uncoupling protein-2	Mitochondria	Adaptive responses to ROS-generating alkylating agent	↑
Hypoxia-induced factor (HIF) system	Transcription factor	Chemoresistance by modulating p53 and nuclear factor-kB	↑
mtTFA, ATF4, ZNF143, Ets-1, AP-2	Transcription factors		↑
SKP2, cyclin D1	Cell cycle related factors		↑
Many ribosomal proteins	Peripheral functions related to apoptosis and DNA repair		↓
Surviving, Xiap	Regulation of anti-apoptosis	Increased apoptosis inhibitors	↑

PDIA: protein disulfide isomerases.

From the above discussions, it can be formulated that a general understanding of the resistance mechanisms against alkylating agents. In tumor cells, resistance to alkylating agents occurs through two basic mechanisms: a) changes in cellular responses leading to increased cell ability to tolerate stress conditions b) acquiring mechanisms to escape apoptosis because of tumor microenvironment, drug efflux via a wide range of drug transporters localized in the cellular membranes, and altered drug metabolism and DNA repair systems. Although numerous mechanisms are found to be associated with drug resistance in cancer so far, we are still far from fully understanding how to overcome drug resistance. The current findings suggest that, appearance of a drug-resistant phenotype is not mediated by a single mechanism. It is clear that drug-resistant phenotype is a result of a network including different cellular pathways. Molecular mechanisms involved in these pathways can be switched on and off, thus temporarily simultaneously active during the development of chemoresistance in patients receiving anticancer therapy. Taken together, there are many gaps that need to be filled in order to solve the complex interactions among molecular factors contributing the development of a drug resistance phenotype.

References

[1]   Harrison, D. J. Molecular mechanisms of drug resistance in tumours. *J. Pathol*, 1995; 175: 7–12.

[2]   Stewart DJ. Tumor and host factors that may limit efficacy of chemotherapy in non-small cell and small cell lung cancer/ *Critical Reviews in Oncology/Hematology*, 2010; 75 :173–234.

[3]   Siddik, ZH. Cisplatin: mode of cytotoxic action and molecular basis of resistance. *Oncogene* , 2003, 22, 7265–7279

[4]   Harada, N; Nagasaki, A; Hata, H; Matsuzaki, H; Matsuno, F; Mitsuya, H. Down-regulation of CD98 in melphalan-resistant myeloma cells with reduced drug uptake. *Acta Haematol.* 2000, 103, 144-151.

[5]   Van Bambeke, F; Michot, J. M; Tulkens, P. M. Antibiotic efflux pumps in eukaryotic cells: occurrence and impact on antibiotic cellular pharmacokinetics, pharmacodynamics and toxicodynamics. *J. Antimicrob. Chemother.* 2003, 51, 1067–1077

[6]   Ueda, K; Cardarelli, C; Gottesman, MM; Pastan, I. Expression of a full-length cDNA for the human 'MDR1' gene confers resistance to colchicine, doxorubicin, and vinblastine *Proc Natl Acad Sci USA* 1987 84: 3004–3008

[7]   Haimeur, A; Conseil G; Deeley RG and Cole SP. The MRP-related and BCRP/ABCG2 multidrug resistance proteins: biology, substrate specificity and regulation. *Curr Drug Metab*, 2004; 5: 21–53.

[8]   Taniguchi, K ;Wada, M; Kohno, K; Nakamura, T; Kawabe, T; Kawakami, M; Kagotani, K; Okumura, K; Akiyama, S; Kuwano, M. A

human canalicular multispecific organic anion transporter (cMOAT) gene is overexpressed in cisplatin-resistant human cancer cell lines with decreased drug accumulation. *Cancer Res.*, 1996;56:4124-4129

[9]   Cole, S.P; Sparks, K.E; Fraser, K; Loe, D.W; Grant, C.E; Wilson, G.M; Deeley, R.G. Pharmacological characterization of multidrug resistant MRP-transfected human tumor cells. *Cancer Res.* 1994,54, 5902–5910.

[10] Ortega, A.; Carretero, J.; Obrador, E.; Estrela, J.M. Tumoricidal activity of endothelium-derived no and the survival of metastatic cells with high GSH and bcl-2 levels. *Nitric. Oxide* 2008, *19*, 107-114.

[11] Yao, K.S.; Godwin, A.K.; Johnson, S.W.; Ozols, R.F.; O'Dwyer, P.J.; Hamilton, T.C. Evidence for altered regulation of gamma-glutamylcysteine synthetase gene expression among cisplatin-sensitive and cisplatin-resistant human ovarian cancer cell lines. *Cancer Res.* 1995, *55*, 4367-4374.

[12] Tew, KD; Monks, A; Barone, L; Rosser, D;Akerman, G; Montali, JA Wheatley, JB; Schmidt, DE Jr. Glutathione-associated enzymes in the human cell lines of the National Cancer Institute Drug Screening Program. *Mol Pharmacol* 1996; 50: 149–159

[13] Fokkema, E; Groen, HJ; Helder, MN; de Vries, EG; Meijer, C.JM216-, JM118-, and cisplatin-induced cytotoxicity in relation to platinum–DNA adduct formation, glutathione levels and p53 status in human tumour cell lines with different sensitivities to cisplatin. *Biochem Pharmacol*, 2002; 63:1989–1996.

[14] Gottesman, MMand Pastan I. 1993, Biochemistry of multidrug resistance mediated by the multidrug transporter. *Ann Rev Biochem*, 62:385–427.

[15] David, J; Waxman. Glutathione 5-Transferases: Role in Alkylating Agent Resistance and Possible Target for Modulation Chemotherapy. *Cancer Research*, 1990;50: 6449-6454.

[16] Hayes, JDand Pulford, DJ. 1995. The glutathione S-transferase supergene family: regulation of GST and the contribution of the isoenzymes to cancer chemoprotection and drug resistance. *Crit. Rev. Biochem. Mol. Biol.*, 30:445–600.

[17] Waxman DJ. Glutathione 5-Transferases: Role in Alkylating Agent Resistance and Possible Target for Modulation Chemotherapy. *Cancer Research*, 1990, 50; 6449-6454.

[18] Lien, S; Larsson, AK and Mannervik, B. The polymorphic human glutathione transferase T1–1, the most efficient glutathione transferase

in the denitrosation and inactivation of the anticancer drug 1,3-bis(2-chloroethyl)-1-nitrosourea. *Biochem Pharmacol*, 2002, 63: 172–191.

[19] Laborde, E. Glutathione transferases as mediators of signaling pathways involved in cell proliferation and cell death. *Cell Death and Differentiation*, 2010; 17: 1373–1380.

[20] Piaggi, S; Raggi, C; Corti, A; Pitzalis, E; Mascherpa, MC; Saviozzi, M; Pompella, A; Casini, AF. Glutathione transferase omega 1-1 (GSTO1-1) plays an anti-apoptotic role in cell resistance to cisplatin toxicity. *Carcinogenesis*, 2010; 31: 804–811.

[21] Miyake, T; Nakayama, T; Naoi, Y; Yamamoto, N; Otani, Y; Kim, SJ; Shimazu, K, Shimomura, A, Maruyama, N; Tamaki, Y; Noguchi, S. GSTP1 expression predicts poor pathological complete response to neoadjuvant chemotherapy in ER-negative breast cancer. *Cancer Sci.* 2012, 103(5):913-20.

[22] Sakamoto, M; Kondo, A; Kawasaki, K; Goto, T; Sakamoto, H; Miyake, K; Koyamatsu, Y; Akiya, T; Iwabuchi, H; Muroya, T. Analysis of gene expression profiles associated with cisplatin resistance in human ovarian cancer cell lines and tissues using cDNA microarray. *Hum Cell.* 2001; 4:305-15.

[23] Liu, G; Yuan, X; Zeng, Z;Tunici, P; Ng, H; Abdulkadir, IR; Lu, L; Irvin, D; Black,KL; Yu, JS. Analysis of gene expression and chemoresistance of CD133+ cancer stem cells in glioblastoma. *Mol Cancer*,2006; 5: 67.

[24] Lo, HW; and Ali-Osman, F. Genetic polymorphism and function of glutathione S-transferases in tumor drug resistance. *Curr Opin Pharmacol*, 2007;7:367-74

[25] Watson, MA; Stewart, RK; Smith, GB; Massey, TE; Bell, DA. Human glutathione S-transferase P1 polymorphisms. *Carcinogenesis.* 1998;19:275-280.

[26] Stoehlmacher J; Park, DJ; Zhang, W; Groshen, S; Tsao-Wei, DD; Yu, MC; Lenz, HJ. Association between glutathione S-transferase P1, T1, and M1 genetic polymorphism and survival of patients with metastatic colorectal cancer. *J Natl Cancer Inst*, 2002,94, 936–942.

[27] Sweeney, C; Ambrosone, CB; Joseph, L; Stone, A; Hutchins, LF; Kadlubar, FF. Coles BF: Association between a glutathione Stransferase A1 promoter polymorphism and survival after breast cancer treatment. Int J Cancer 2003, 103:810-814. *Current Opinion in Pharmacology*, 2007; 7:367–374.

[28] Dylla, SJ; Beviglia, L; Park, I-K; Chartie,r C; Raval, J; Ngan, L; Pickell, K; Aguilar, J; Lazetic, S; Smith-Berdan, S; Clarke, MF; Hoey, T;

Lewicki, J; Gurney, AL. (2008) Colorectal Cancer Stem Cells Are Enriched in Xenogeneic Tumors Following Chemotherapy. *PLoS ONE* 3(6): e2428. doi:10.1371/journal.pone.0002428

[29] Sladek, NE; Kollander, R; Sreerama, L; Kiang, DT; Cellular levels of aldehyde dehydrogenases (ALDH1A1 and ALDH3A1) as predictors of therapeutic responses to cyclophosphamide-based chemotherapy of breast cancer: a retrospective study. Rational individualization of oxazaphosphorine based cancer chemotherapeutic regimens. *Cancer Chemother Pharmacol* 2002, 49:309–321.

[30] Helsby, NA; Hui, CY; Goldthorpe, MA; Coller, JK; Soh, MC; Gow, PJ; De Zoysa, JZ; and Tingle, MD (2010). The combined impact of CYP2C19 and CYP2B6 pharmacogenetics on cyclophosphamide bioactivation. *B J Clin Pharmacol*; 70, 844-853.

[31] Bray, J; Sludden, J; Griffin, J; Cole, M; Verrill, M; Jamieson, D; and Boddy, AV. Influence of pharmacogenetics on response and toxicity in breast cancer patients treated with doxorubicin and cyclophosphamide. *Br J Cancer*, 2010, 102, 1003-1009.

[32] Efferth, T; V, Manfred. Pharmacogenetics for individualized cancer chemotherapy. *Pharmacology and Therapeutics*, 2005, 107, 155 – 176.

[33] Pegg, AE. Mammalian O6-alkylguanine-DNA alkyltransferase: regulation and importance in response to alkylating carcinogenic and therapeutic agents. *Cancer Res*, 1990; 50: 6119-29.

[34] Middleton, M R; Margison, G P. Improvement of chemotherapy efficacy by inactivation of a DNA-repair pathway. *The Lancet Oncology*, 2003; 4, 37–44.

[35] Pegg, AE; Dolan, ME; Moschel, RC. Structure, function, and inhibition of O6-alkylguanine-DNA alkyltransferase. *Prog Nucleic Acid Res Mol Biol*, 1995; 51:167-223.

[36] Baer, JC; Freeman, AA; Newlands, ES; Watson, AJ; Rafferty, JA; Margison, GP. Depletion of O^6-alkylguanine-DNA alkyltransferase correlates with potentiation of temozolomide and CCNU toxicity in human tumour cells. *Br J Cancer*. 1993;67:1299–302.

[37] Friedman, HS; Dolan, ME; Pegg, AE; Marcelli, S; Keir, S; Catino, JJ; Bigner, DD; Schold, SC Jr. Activity of temozolomide in the treatment of central nervous system tumor xenografts. *Cancer Res*, 1995; 55: 2853–2857.

[38] Glassner, BJ; Weeda, G; Allan, JM; Broekhof, JL; Carls, NH; Donker, I; Engelward, BP; Hampson, RJ; Hersmus, R; Hickman, MJ; Roth, RB; Warren, HB; Wu, MM; Hoeijmakers, JH; Samson, LD. DNA repair

methyltransferase (MGMT) knockout mice are sensitive to the lethal effects of chemotherapeutic alkylating agents. *Mutagenesis*, 1999; 14:339–347.

[39] Zhou, ZQ; Manguino, D; Kewitt, K; Intano, GW; McMahan, CA; Herbert, DC; Hanes, M; Reddick, R; Ikeno, Y; Walter, CA.. Spontaneous hepatocellular carcinoma is reduced in transgenic mice overexpressing human O6 methylguanine-DNA methyltransferase. *Proc Natl Acad Sci USA* 2001, 98, 12566–12571.

[40] Hegi, ME; Diserens, AC; Godard, S; Dietrich, PY; Regli, L; Ostermann, S; Otten, P; Van Melle, G; de Tribolet, N; Stupp, R. Clinical trial substantiates the predictivevalue of O-6-methylguanine-DNA methyltransferase promoter methylation in glioblastoma patients treated with temozolomide. *Clin Cancer Res*, 2004, 10:1871–1874.

[41] Wedge, SR; Porteous, JK; Newlands ES. 3-aminobenzamide and/or O^6-benzylguanine evaluated as an adjuvant to temozolomide or BCNU treatment in cell lines of variable mismatch repair status and O6-alkylguanine-DNA alkyltransferase activity. *Br J Cancer* 1996;74:1030–6.

[42] Gerson, SL. MGMT: its role in cancer aetiology and cancer therapeutics. *Nat Rev Cancer*, 2004; 4:296-307.

[43] Hotta, T; Saito, Y; Fujita, H; Mikami ,T; Kurisu, K; Kiya, K; Uozumi, T; Isowa, G; Ishizaki, K; Ikenaga, M. O6-alkylguanine-DNA alkyltransferase activity of human malignant glioma and its clinical implications. *J Neuro oncol*, 1994,21:135-40.

[44] Fan, S; El-Deity, W. S; Bae, I; Freeman, 3; Jondle, D; Bhatia, K; Fomace, A. J; Magrath, I; Kohn, K. W; and O'Connor, M. p53 gene mutations are associated with decreased sensitivity of human lymphoma cells to DNA damaging agents. *Cancer Res*, 1994; 54: 5824-5830.

[45] Oliva, CR; Moellering, DR; Gillespie, GY;Griguer, CE. (2011) Acquisition of Chemoresistance in Gliomas Is Associated with Increased Mitochondrial Coupling and Decreased ROS Production. *PLoS ONE* 6(9): e24665. doi:10.1371/journal.pone.0024665

[46] Esteller, M; Herman, JG. Generating mutations but providing chemosensitivity: the role of O^6-methylguanine DNA methyltransferase in human cancer. *Oncogene*, 2004;23:1–8.

[47] Fang, Q; Loktionova, N. A; Moschel, R. C; Javanmard, S; Pauly, G. T;and Pegg, A. E. Differential in activation of polymorphic variants of human O6-alkylguanine-DNA alkyltransferase. *Biochem. Pharmacol*, 2008; 75: 618–626.

[48] Herfarth, KK; Brent, TP; Danam, RP; Remack, JS; Kodner, IJ; Wells, SA; Jr, Goodfellow, PJ. A specific CpG methylation pattern of the MGMT promoter region associated with reduced MGMT expression in primary colorectal cancers,1999;24:90-8.

[49] Wolf, P; Hu, YC; Doffek, K; Sidransky, D; Ahrendt, SA. O(6)-Methylguanine-DNA methyltransferase promoter hypermethylation shifts the p53 mutational spectrum in non-small cell lung cancer. *Cancer Res*, 2001, 61, 8113-8117.

[50] Monika, E; Liu, HL; Herman, JG; Stupp, R; Wick ,W; Weller, M; Mehta, MP; and Gilbert, MR. Correlation of O^6-Methylguanine Methyltransferase (MGMT) Promoter Methylation With Clinical Outcomes in Glioblastoma and Clinical Strategies to Modulate MGMT Activity. *J Clin Oncol*, 2008; 26:4189-4199.

[51] Kesari, S; Schiff, D; Drappatz, J; LaFrankie, D; Doherty, L; Macklin, E.A; Muzikan-sky, A; Santagata, S; Ligon, K.L; Norden, A.D; Ciampa, A; Bradshaw, J; Levy, B; Radakovic, G., Ramakrishna, N., Black, P.M; Wen, P.Y. Phase II study of protracted daily temozolomide for low-grade gliomas in adults. *Clin. Cancer. Res.*, 2009;15: 330–337.

[52] Redmond, K.M; Wilson, T.R; Johnston, P.G; Longley, D.B. Resistance mechanisms to cancer chemotherapy. *Front. Biosci*, 2008, 13; 5138–5154.

[53] D'Amours, D; Desnoyers, S; D'Silva, I; and Poirier, G.G. Poly(ADP-ribosyl)ation reactions in the regulation of nuclear functions. *Biochem. J*, 1999; 342 : 249-268.

[54] Kim, M.Y; Mauro, S; Gevry, N; Lis, J.T; and Kraus, W.L. NAD^+-dependent modulation of chromatin structure and transcription by nucleosome binding properties of PARP-1. *Cell*, 2004; 119: 803-814

[55] Masson, M; Niedergang, C; Schreiber, V; Muller, S; Menissier de Murcia, J and de Murcia, G. XRCC1 is specifically associated with poly(ADP-ribose) polymerase and negatively regulates its activity following DNA damage. *Mol. Cell. Biol*, 1998;18: 3563-3571

[56] Masutani, M; Nozaki, T; Nakamoto, K; Nakagama, H; Suzuki H; Kusuoka, O; Tsutsumi, M; Sugimura, T. The response of Parp knockout mice against DNA damaging agents. *Mutat Res*. 2000, 462, 159-66.

[57] Selvakumaran, M; Pisarcik, DA; Bao, R; Yeung, AT; Hamilton, TC. Enhanced cisplatin cytotoxicity by disturbing the nucleotide excision repair pathway in ovarian cancer cell lines. *Cancer Res*, 2003, 63, 1311-1316.

[58] Lainie, P; Thomas, CM; Hamilton and Russell J Schilder. Platinum Resistance: The Role of DNA Repair Pathways. *Clin Cancer Res* 2008; 14: 1291-1295.

[59] Reed, E. Platinum-DNA adduct, nucleotide excision repair and platinum based anti-cancer chemotherapy. *Cancer Treat Rev*, 1998; 24: 331–344.

[60] Boyer, J; McLean, EG; Aroori, S; Wilson, P; McCulla, A; Carey, PD; Longley, DB; Johnston, PG. Characterization of p53 wild-type and null isogenic colorectal cancer cell lines resistant to 5-fluorouracil, oxaliplatin, and irinotecan. *Clin Cancer Res*. 2004; 10: 2158–2167

[61] Hector, S; Bolanowska-Higdon, W; Zdanowicz, J; Hitt, S; Pendyala, L. In vitro studies on the mechanisms of oxaliplatin resistance. *Cancer Chemother Pharmacol*, 2001; 48: 398–406.

[62] Dabholkar, M; Vionnet, J; Bostick-Bruton, F; Yu, JJ; Reed, E. Messenger RNA levels of XPAC and ERCC1 in ovarian cancer tissue correlate with response to platinum-based chemotherapy. *J Clin Invest*, 1994; 94: 703–708

[63] Lord, RV; Brabender, J; Gandara, D ; Alberola, V; Camps, C; Domine, M; Cardenal, F; Sánchez, JM; Gumerlock, PH; Tarón, M; Sánchez, JJ; Danenberg, KD; Danenberg, PV; Rosell, R. Low ERCC1 expression correlates with prolonged survival after cisplatin plus gemcitabine chemotherapy in non-small cell lung cancer. *Clin Cancer Res*, 2002; 8: 2286–2291.

[64] Chen, HY; Shao, CJ; Chen, FR; Kwan, AL; Chen, ZP. Role of ERCC1 promoter hypermethylation in drug resistance to cisplatin in human gliomas. *Int J Cancer*, 2010,126:1944-54.

[65] Wu, Y; Xiao, Y; Ding, X; Zhuo, Y; Ren, P; Zhou, C; Zhou, J. A miR-200b/200c/429-Binding Site Polymorphism in the 39 Untranslated Region of the AP-2a Gene Is Associated with Cisplatin Resistance. *PLoS ONE*, 2011, 6(12): e29043. doi:10.1371/journal.pone.0029043

[66] Fink, D; Aebi, D; Howell, SB. The role of DNA mismatch repair in drug resistance. *Clin Cancer Res*, 1998; 4: 1–6.

[67] Lage, H; Dietel, M. Involvement of the DNA mismatch repair system in antineoplastic drug resistance. *J Cancer Res ClinOncol*,1999; 125:156-165.

[68] Karran, P; Mechanisms of tolerance to DNA damaging therapeutic drugs, *Carcinogenesis*, 2001; 22 :1931–1937.

[69] Plumb, JA; Strathdee, G; Sludden, J; Kaye, SB; Brown, R. Reversal of drug resistance in human tumor xenografts by 29-deoxy-5-azacytidine-

induced demethylation of the hMLH1 gene promoter. *Cancer Res*, 2000; 60:6039–6044.

[70] Yip, S; Miao, J; Cahill, DP; Iafrate, AJ; Aldape, K; Nutt, CL; and Louis, DN. MSH6 Mutations Arise in Glioblastomas during Temozolomide Therapy and Mediate Temozolomide Resistance *Clin Cancer Res* 2009, 5, 4622-4629

[71] Eijdems, EWHM; De Haas, M; Timmermann, AJ; Van der Schans, GP; Kamst, E; De Nooji, J; Astaldi-Ricotti, GCB; Bors, t P; Baas, F. Reduced topoisomerase I activity in multidrug-resistant human non-small cell lung cancer cell lines. *Br J Cancer*, 1985; 71: 40-47.

[72] Dingemans, AM; Witlox, MA; Stallaert, RA; van der Valk, P; Postmus, PE; Giaccone, G. Expression of DNA topoisomerase II alpha and topoisomerase II beta genes predicts survival and response to chemotherapy in patients with small cell lung cancer. *Clin Cancer Res*, 1999; 5: 2048-2058.

[73] Pu, QQ; Bezwoda, WR. 1999. Induction of alkylator (melphalan) resistance in HL60 cells is accompanied by increased levels of topoisomerase II expression and function. *Mol Pharmacol*, 56; 147-153.

[74] Henkels, KM and Turchi, JJ. Induction of apoptosis in cisplatin-sensitive and -resistant human ovarian cancer cell lines. *Cancer Res*, 1997; 57: 4488–4492

[75] Hamano, R; Miyata, H; Yamasaki, M; Kurokawa, Y; Hara, J Moon, JH; Nakajima, K; Takiguchi, S; Fujiwara, Y; Mori, M; Doki ,Y. Overexpression of miR-200c Induces Chemoresistance in Esophageal Cancers Mediated Through Activation of the Akt Signaling Pathway. *Clin Cancer Res*, 2011; 17: 3029–3038.

[76] Danilov, AV; Neupane, D; Nagaraja, AS; Feofanova, EV; Humphries, LA; DiRenzo, J; Korc, M. DeltaNp63alpha-mediated induction of epidermal growth factor receptor promotes pancreatic cancer cell growth and chemoresistance. *PloSOne* 2011;6(10):e26815.

[77] Shain, KH; Landowski, TH; Dalton, WS. Adhesion-mediated intracellular redistribution of c-Fas-associated death domain-like IL-1-converting enzyme like inhibitory protein-long confers resistance to CD95-induced apoptosis in hematopoietic cancer cell lines. *J. Immunol*, 2002; 168: 2544–2553.

[78] Badie, B; Kramar, MH; Lau, R; Boothman, DA; Economou, JS; Black, KL. Adenovirus-mediated p53 gene delivery potentiates the radiation-induced growth inhibition of experimental brain tumors. *J Neuro oncol.* 1998:217-22.

[79] Brown, R; Clugston, C; Bums, P; Edlin, A; Vasey, P; Vojtesek. B; Kaye, S. B. Increased accumulation of p53 protein in cisplatin-resistant ovarian cell lines. *Int. J. Cancer*, 1993, 55: 678-684.

[80] Kirsch, Dand Kastan, M. 1998. Tumor-suppressor p53: implications for tumor development and prognosis. *J Clin Oncol;* 16:3158.

[81] Yang, XK; Zheng, F; Chen, JH; Gao, QL; Lu, YP; Wang, SX; Wang, CY and a, Ma. D Relationship between expression of apoptosis-associated proteins and caspase-3 activity in cisplatin-resistant human ovarian cancer cell line. *Ai Zheng*, 2002; 21 1288–1291.

[82] Vegran, F; Boidot, R; Oudin, C; Riedinger, JM; Bonnetain, F; Lizard-Nacol, S. Overexpression of caspase-3s splice variant in locally advanced breast carcinoma is associated with poor response to neoadjuvant chemotherapy. *Clin Cancer Res* 2006, 12:5794-5800.

[83] Amaravadi, RK; Yu, D; Lum, JJ; Bui, T; Christophorou; MA, Evan; GI Thomas-Tikhonenko, A; Thompson CB. Autophagy inhibition enhances therapy-induced apoptosis in a Myc-induced model of lymphoma. *J Clin Invest* 2007;117:326–36.

[84] Jun, F; Zhi-gang, L; Xiao-mei, L; Fu-rong, C; Hong-liu, S; Jesse Chung-sean, P; NG Ho-keung ; Zhong-ping, C. Glioblastoma stem cells resistant to temozolomide-induced autophagy. *Chinese Medical Journal*, 2009, 122, 1255-1259

[85] Kondo, Y; Kanzawa, T; Sawaya, R; Kondo, S. The role of autophagy in cancer development and response to therapy. *Nat Rev Cancer,* 2005;5:726–734.

[86] Liang, XH; Jackson, S; Seaman, M; Brown, K; mpkes, B; Hibshoosh, H; Levine B. Induction of autophagy and inhibition of tumorigenesis by beclin 1. *Nature*, 1999; 402: 672–676.

[87] Kanzawa, T; Germano, IM; Komata, T; Ito, H; Kondo, Y; Kondo, S. Role of autophagy in temozolomide induced cytotoxicity for malignant glioma cells. *Cell Death Differ*, 2004, 11, 448–457.

[88] Ma, X; Piao, S; Wang, D; Mcafee, QW; Nathanson, KL; Lum, JJ; Li, LZ; and Amaravadi, RK. Measurements of Tumor Cell Autophagy Predict Invasiveness, Resistance to Chemotherapy, and Survival in Melanoma. *Clin Cancer Res*, 2011; *17:* 3478

[89] Volinia, S; Calin, GA; Liu C, et al. A microRNA expression signature of human solid tumors defines cancer gene targets. *Proc Natl Acad Sci USA* 2006;103 (7):2257–61.

[90] Teicher, BA; Herman, TS; Holden, SA; Wang YY, Pfeffer, MR; Crawford, JW; Frei E 3rd. Tumor resistance to alkylating agents

conferred by mechanisms operative only in vivo. *Science*, 1990; 247 : 1457 – 61 .

[91] Maubant, S; Cruet-Hennequart, S; Poulain L; Carreiras, F; Sichel, F; Luis, J; Staedel, C; Gauduchon, P. Altered adhesion properties and alphav integrin expression in a cisplatin-resistant human ovarian carcinoma cell line. *Int J Cancer* 2002; 97:186–194.

[92] Correia, ALand Bissell, MJ 2012. The tumor microenvironment is a dominant force in multidrug resistance. *Drug Resist Updat*. 15,39-49.

[93] Azab, AK; Quang, P; Azab, F; Pitsillides, C; Thompson, B; Chonghaile, T; Patton, JT; Maiso, P; Monrose, V; Sacco, A; Ngo, HT; Flores, LM; Lin, CP; Magnani, JL; Kung, AL; Letai, A; Carrasco, R; Roccaro, AM; Ghobrial, IM.P-selecting glycoprotein ligand regulates the interaction of multiple myeloma cells with the bone marrow microenvironment. *Blood*. 2012 , 119:1468-1478.

[94] Croix, BS; Rak, JW; Kapitain, S; Sheehan, C; Graham, CH; Kerbel, RS. Reversal by hyaluronidase of adhesion-dependent multicellular drug resistance in mammary carcinoma cells. *J Natl Cancer Inst*, 1996; 88:1285-1296.

[95] Croix, B; Florenes, VA; Rak, JW; Flanagan, M; Bhattacharya, N; Slingerland, JM; Kerbel, RS: Impact of the cyclin-dependent kinase inhibitor p27kip1 on resistance of tumor cells to anticancer agents. *Nature Med*, 1996; 2:1204,

[96] Damiano, JS; Hazlehurst, LA; Dalton, WS. Cell adhesion mediated drug resistance (CAM-DR) protects the K562 chronic yelogenous leukemia cell line from apoptosis induced by BCR/ABL inhibition, cytotoxic drugs, and -irradiation. *Leukemia* (Baltimore), 2001; 15: 1232–9.

[97] Hazlehurst, LA; Enkemann, SA; Beam, CA; Argilagos, RF; Painter, J; Shain, KH; Saporta, S; Boulware, D; Moscinski, L; Alsina, M; Dalton, WS. Genotypic and phenotypic comparisons of de novo and acquired melphalan resistance in an isogenic multiple myeloma cell line model. *Cancer Res*, 2003;63:7900-6.

[98] Borsellino, N; Belldegrun, A; and Bonavida, B. Endogenous interleukin 6 is a resistance factor for *cis*-diamminedichloroplatinum and etoposide-mediated cytotoxicity of human prostate carcinoma cell lines. *Cancer Res*, 1995; *55:* 4633–4639,

[99] Rossi, J.F; Fegueux, N; Lu, Z.Y; Legouffe, E; Exbrayat, C; Bozonnat, M.C; Navarro, R; Lopez, E., Quittet, P; Daures, J.P; Rouille, V; Kanouni, T; Widjenes, J., Klein, B. Optimizing the use of anti-interleukin-6 monoclonal antibody with dexamethasone and 140 mg/m2

of melphalan in multiple myeloma: results of a pilot study including biological aspects. *Bone Marrow Transplantation.* 2005; 36: 771–779.

[100] Clarke, MF; Dick, JE; Dirks, PB Eaves, CJ; Jamieson, CH; Jones, DL; Visvader, J; Weissman, IL; Wahl, GM. Cancer Stem Cells— Perspectives on Current Status and Future Directions: AACR Workshop on Cancer Stem Cells. *Cancer Res.* 2006; 66:9339–9344.

[101] Dean, M; Fojo, T; Bates, S. Tumour stem cells and drug resistance. Nat Rev Cancer, 2005; 5: 275–84.

[102] Eramo, A; Ricci-Vitiani, L; Zeuner, A; Pallini, R; Lotti, F; Sette, G; Pilozzi, E; Larocca, LM; Peschle, C; De Maria, R. Chemotherapy resistance of glioblastoma stem cells. *Cell Death Differ*, 2006; 13:1238-1241.

[103] Kang, MK; Kang, SK. Tumorigenesis of chemotherapeutic drug-resistant cancer stem-like cells in brain glioma. *Stem Cells Dev*, 2007; 16: 837–847.

[104] Singh, SK; Hawkins, C; Clarke, ID; Squire, JA; Bayani, J; Hide, T; Henkelman, RM; Cusimano, MD; Dirks PB. Identification of human brain tumour initiating cells. *Nature*, 2004;432: 396–401.

[105] Diehn, M; Cho, RW; Lobo, NA; Kalisky, T; Dorie, MJ; Kulp, AN; Qian, D; Lam, JS; Ailles, LE; Wong, M; Joshua, B; Kaplan, MJ; Wapnir, I; Dirbas, F; Somlo, G; Garberoglio, C; Paz, B; Shen, J; Lau ,SK; Quake, SR; Brown, JM; Weissman, IL and Clarke, MF. Association of reactive oxygen species levels and radioresistance in cancer stem cells. *Nature.* 2009 9, 458, 780-783.

[106] Stupp, R; Hegi, ME. Targeting brain-tumor stem cells. *Nature Biotechnology*, 2007; 25: 193-194.

[107] Blower, PE; Chung, J. Verducci; JS, Lin; S, Park; JK, Dai; Z, Liu; CG, Schmittgen; TD, Reinhold; WC, Croce; CM, Weinstein; JN, Sadee W. MicroRNAs modulate the chemosensitivity of tumor cells. *Mol Cancer Ther.* 2008;7:1–9.

[108] Blower, PE; Verducci, JS; Lin, S; Park, JK; Dai, Z; Liu, CG; Schmittgen, TD; Reinhold, WC; Croce, CM; Weinstein, JN; Sadee, W. microRNA expression profiles for the NCI-60 cancer cell panel. *Mol Cancer Ther* 2007;6:1483–591.

[109] Calin, G.A. and Croce, C.M. microRNA signatures in human cancers. *Nature*, 2006;6:857–66.

[110] Giovannetti, E; Erozenci, A; Smit, J; Romano, Danesi; Peters GJ. Molecular mechanisms underlying the role of microRNAs (miRNAs) in

anticancer drug resistance and implications for clinical practice. *Critical Reviews in Oncology/Hematology*, 2012; 81: 103–122

[111] Shi, L; Chen, C; Yang, J; Pan, T; Zhang, S; Wang, Z. MiR-21 protected human glioblastoma U87MG cells from chemotherapeutic drug temozolomide induced apoptosis by decreasing Bax/Bcl-2 ratio and caspase-3 activity. *Brain Res*, 2010,1352:255–264

[112] Ujifuku, K; Mitsutake, N; Takakura, S; Matsuse, M; Saenko, V; Suzuki, K; Hayashi, K; Matsuo, T; Kamada, K; Nagata, I; Yamashita, S. miR-195, miR-455-3p and miR-10a (*) are implicated in acquired temozolomide resistance in glioblastoma multiforme cells. *Cancer Lett.* 2010, 28, 296, 241-248.

[113] Lee, JW; Park, YA; Choi, JJ; Lee, YY; Kim, CJ; Choi, C; Kim, TJ; Lee, NW; Kim, BG; Bae, DS. (2011) The expression of the miRNA-200 family in endometrial endometrioid carcinoma. *Gynecol Oncol* 120: 56–62.

[114] Hamano, R; Miyata, H; Yamasaki, M; Kurokawa, Y; Hara, J Moon, JH; Nakajima, K; Takiguchi, S; Fujiwara, Y; Mori, M; Doki ,Y. Overexpression of miR-200c Induces Chemoresistance in Esophageal Cancers Mediated Through Activation of the Akt Signaling Pathway. *Clin Cancer Res*, 2011; 17: 3029–3038.

[115] Blower, PE; Chung, J. Verducci; JS, Lin; S, Park; JK, Dai; Z, Liu; CG, Schmittgen; TD, Reinhold; WC, Croce ;CM, Weinstein; JN, Sadee W. MicroRNAs modulate the chemosensitivity of tumor cells. *Mol Cancer Ther.* 2008;7:1–9.

[116] Wu, Y; Xiao, Y; Ding, X; Zhuo, Y; Ren, P; Zhou, C; Zhou, J. A miR-200b/200c/429-Binding Site Polymorphism in the 39 Untranslated Region of the AP-2a Gene Is Associated with Cisplatin Resistance. *PLoS ONE*, 2011, 6(12): e29043. doi:10.1371/journal.pone.0029043

[117] Chavez, JD; Hoopmann, MR; Weisbrod, CR; Takara, K; Bruce, JE. (2011) Quantitative Proteomic and Interaction Network Analysis of Cisplatin Resistance in HeLa Cells. *PLoS ONE* 6(5): e19892. doi:10.1371/journal.pone.0019892.

In: Alkylating Agents ...   ISBN: 978-1-62618-487-9
Editor: Yildiz Dincer   © 2013 Nova Science Publishers, Inc.

Chapter V

Alkylating Agents and Treatment of Gliomas

*Tsuyoshi Fukushima**

Section of Oncopathology and Regenerative Biology,
Department of Pathology, Faculty of Medicine,
University of Miyazaki, Miyazaki, Japan

Abstract

Nitrosoureas have been commonly used for the treatment of
malignant gliomas since the 1970s. However, the prognosis of patients
with malignant gliomas remains extremely poor despite the fact that
multidisciplinary approaches involving surgery, chemotherapy, and
radiotherapy have been used for several decades. Recently, the novel
alkylating agent temozolomide (TMZ) was shown to improve the survival
of patients with malignant gliomas (including glioblastomas) in many
clinical studies and has become one of the standard modalities for
treatment of newly diagnosed and recurrent malignant gliomas.
Temozolomide is a prodrug that can be orally administered and is
hydrolytically processed in the blood to yield the methyldiazonium

* Correspondence to: Tsuyoshi Fukushima, MD, PhD, Section of Oncopathology and
  Regenerative Biology, Department of Pathology, Faculty of Medicine, University of
  Miyazaki, 5200 Kihara, Kiyotake, Miyazaki 889-1692, Japan, Telephone: +81 985 85 2809;
  Fax: +81 985 85 6003, E-mail: fukuchan@med.miyazaki-u.ac.jp

cation, which has DNA methylating activity. Patients can receive ambulatory treatment with TMZ because of its oral administration route and minimal side effects. The expression level of the DNA repair enzyme O6-methylguanine-DNA methyltransferase (MGMT) is the most important factor for a favorable outcome in patients treated with TMZ as well as those treated with nitrosoureas, and the epigenetic silencing of *MGMT* is the strongest predictive marker. The treatment course for patients with tumors lacking *MGMT* promoter methylation is unknown, and recurrence is unavoidable even in patients with TMZ-sensitive glioblastoma. While TMZ has provided a significant survival benefit, innovative modalities that can be combined with TMZ and radiotherapy are still required. In this chapter, we review the history and chemistry of alkylating agents for the treatment of malignant gliomas. In particular, we focus on TMZ and its effects on tumor cells. Furthermore, chemoresistance to TMZ and current chemotherapies used for the treatment of malignant gliomas are discussed.

Introduction

Gliomas represent the most common primary tumors of the adult central nervous system (CNS). Despite innovations in neurosurgical devices and techniques, the development of antineoplastic drugs and molecular target drugs, and advances in radiotherapy over the past decades, malignant gliomas—especially glioblastoma (glioblastoma multiforme, GBM)—are still fatal diseases. The World Health Organization (WHO) grading system is widely accepted as a tool for predicting the biological behavior of CNS neoplasms including gliomas. Anaplastic astrocytoma, anaplastic oligodendroglioma, and anaplastic oligoastrocytoma are classified as grade III, and GBM is classified as grade IV. Alkylating agents, especially nitrosoureas such as lomustine (CCNU), have been used to treat high-grade gliomas or malignant gliomas (Grades III and IV). Optionally, subsets of unresectable grade II gliomas could be adaptation diseases. The standard of treatment for malignant gliomas is surgery followed by chemotherapy with radiotherapy. Optionally, boost radiotherapy or chemotherapy is added, and stereotactic radiotherapy or chemotherapy is performed as a salvage therapy upon recurrence/regrowth [1, 2, 3]. Gross total resection is directly associated with longer survival [4], and a randomized trial showed that fluorescence-guided maximum surgical resection improves 6-month progression-free survival [5]. However, patients with malignant gliomas cannot be cured by surgery alone regardless of the surgical technique employed. In the late 1970s, it was reported that the addition of radiotherapy to surgery was more beneficial than surgery alone for patients with malignant gliomas [6, 7]. Although chemotherapy was mainly combined with alkylating agents during this era, there was controversy regarding the benefit of chemotherapy for patients with malignant gliomas. PCV-3, which is a combination of procarbazine, CCNU, and vincristine, is the most common chemotherapy regimen and conferred improved survival and increased time to progression in patients with anaplastic astrocytoma in comparison with the outcomes obtained using a single agent and radiotherapy alone [8]. However, no regimen for the treatment of GBM showed a significant benefit relative to radiotherapy alone until 2003. The Neuro-Oncology Working Group of the German Cancer Society (NOA) reported that a nimustine (ACNU)-based regimen caused a significant improvement in median survival relative to radiotherapy alone [9]. Furthermore, Stupp et al. reported that a novel alkylating agent, temozolomide (TMZ), improved survival in GBM when administered with concomitant radiotherapy in phase II and III studies [10, 11]. TMZ has been regarded as a well-tolerated oral alkylating agent, and the favorable results of clinical studies led to the widespread use of TMZ [12, 13]. The mammalian DNA repair protein O6-methylguanine-DNA methyltransferase (MGMT) has been implicated in the resistance of tumor cells to alkylating agents [14]. To date, many clinical trials have aimed to reduce TMZ resistance. In this chapter, we review the use of alkylating agents, including TMZ, in the treatment of malignant gliomas, their mechanism of antiglioma action, and the findings of clinical trials. Current concepts of chemotherapy in the context of a multidisciplinary approach to the treatment of malignant gliomas are also discussed.

Alkylating Agents for the Treatment of Brain Tumors

Alkylating agents contribute alkyl groups to DNA causing apoptosis of tumor cells. These agents include nitrogen mustards, ethyleneimines and methylmelamines, methylhydrazine derivatives, alkyl sulfonates, nitrosoureas, and triazenes [15]. Nitrosoureas such as carmustine (BCNU), ACNU, CCNU, semustine (methyl-CCNU), and ranimustine(MCNU) are lipophilic and can pass through the blood-brain barrier, which is one reason why they are the most widely used agents for the treatment of brain tumors. The nitrosoureas exert cytotoxicity via spontaneous breakdown to an alkylating intermediate, the 2-chloroethyl diazoniumion, which alkylates guanine residues in DNA. One of the triazenes, TMZ, also targets guanine and induces methylation. Moreover, the methylhydrazine derivative procarbabazine also induces guanine methylation and is a component of the PCV-3 regimen. The structural formulas of these agents are shown in Figure 1. The other component of PCV-3, vincristine, is not an alkylating agent but rather a vinca alkaloid, which is a natural cell cycle-specific compound.

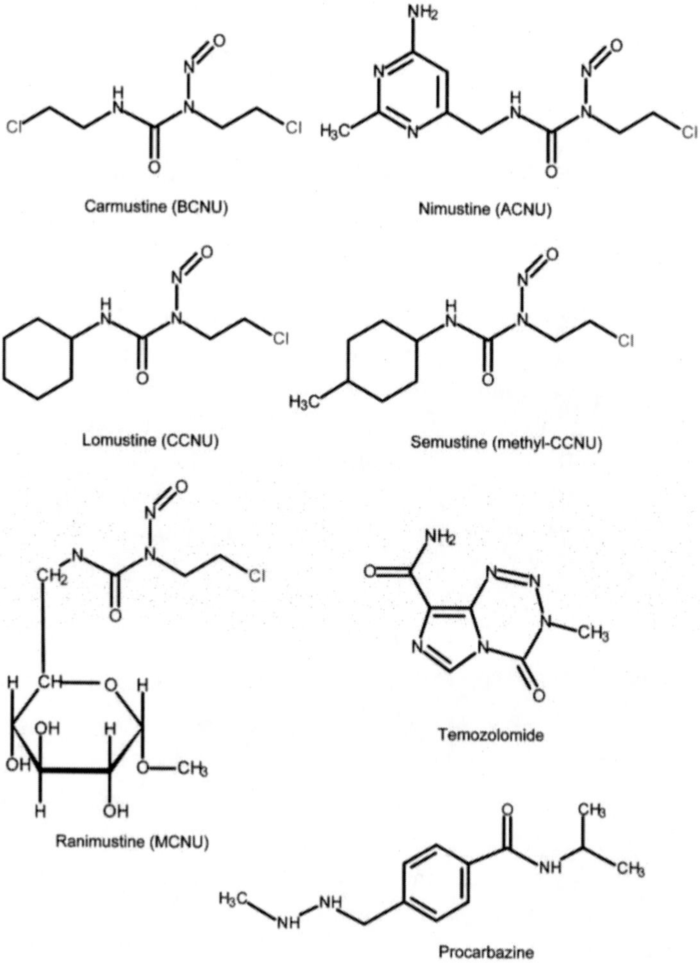

Figure 1. Structural formulae of alkylating agents.

TMZ is orally administered, while the other components are systemically administered. The Brain Tumor Study Group revealed that intra-arterial administration of BCNU did not yield more favorable results than intravenous administration [16]. Recently, intraoperative local treatment with Gliadel (BCNU) wafers was approved, and malignant glioma patients treated with BCNU wafers at the initial surgery in combination with radiation therapy demonstrated a survival advantage compared with those treated with placebo [17].

Prognosis of GBM and Therapeutic Effects of Chemoradiotherapy

The median survival durations of anaplastic astrocytoma patients treated with PCV-3 and BCNU were 157 weeks and 82.1 weeks, respectively. The time to progression was also doubled. However, there was no statistically significant difference in the survival duration of GBM patients regardless of treatment (median, 50.4 weeks with PCV and 57.4 weeks with BCNU) [8, 18]. Despite these results, PCV-3 has been the most extensively used treatment for malignant glioma for a long time. Recent studies have demonstrated that loss of heterozygosity (LOH) on chromosomes 1p and 19q in patients with anaplastic oligodendroglioma predicts sensitivity to chemotherapy and better overall survival [19, 20]. PCV-3 is preferably used in patients who have malignant gliomas with oligodendroglial components. The NOA reported the beneficial effects of ACNU-based chemotherapy in the NOA-1 trial. In phase III of this trial, ACNU plus teniposide (VM26) resulted in a median survival of 17.3 months in 154 GBM patients, and ACNU plus cytosine arabinoside (ara-C) in addition to radiotherapy resulted in a median survival of 15.7 months in 147 GBM patients. These survival benefits are more favorable than those described in any other phase III trial, including later TMZ studies [9, 21]. In the phase III trial reported by the European Organization for Research and Treatment of Cancer (EORTC) and the National Cancer Institute of Canada Clinical Trials Group (NCIC CTG), a combined initial treatment for glioblastoma, including TMZ and radiotherapy, improved survival in comparison with radiotherapy alone over a 5-year follow-up period [11]. The overall survival rate at 5 years was 9.8% (of 287 GBM patients) with TMZ and radiotherapy and 1.9% (of 286 GBM patients) with radiotherapy alone. The median survival duration was 14.6 months with combined therapy and

12.1 months with radiotherapy alone. It is noteworthy that patients with a methylated MGMT promoter who were treated with TMZ and radiotherapy had a longer progression-free survival (23.4 months) [11].

Mechanism of Anticancer Action of TMZ

Similar to dacarbazine (DTIC), TMZ is a triazene. Stevens et al. synthesized TMZ as an analogue of mitozolomide, one of the antitumor imidazotetrazines, in the 1980s [22]. Although mitozolomide showed severe myelosuppression in a phase I study [23], TMZ (a 3-methyl derivative of mitozolomide) was less toxic than mitozolomide and exhibited broad-spectrum activity in mouse tumors [24]. TMZ was also well tolerated and effective in a phase I study [25].

Orally administered TMZ is converted to 5-(3-methyltriazen-1-yl) imidazole-4-carboximide (MTIC) in water/blood with little or no enzymatic component [26, 27]. MTIC is also an intermediate of DTIC degradation and is broken down to the methyldiazonium cation and 5-aminoimidazole-4-carboxamide (AIC) [27]. Although AIC is excreted via the kidneys, the methyldiazonium cation delivers a methyl group to DNA [27]. This methyl group is transferred to the oxygen atom at the 6th position of guanine to generate O6-methylguanine. O6-methylguanine mispairs with thymine instead of cytosine during DNA replication. The O6-methylguanine: thymine mispair can be recognized by the post-replication mismatch repair system, which removes the daughter strand along with the thymine, leaving the O6-methylguanine to again pair with thymine during gap filling. If replication of the gapped DNA occurs, double strand breaks can be formed that result in cell death unless they are repaired by recombination repair pathways. The generation of a methylating intermediate from TMZ is shown in Figure 2. Because this cytotoxicity is replication-dependent, methylating agents including TMZ are more effective in tumor cells than in quiescent cells [26, 27].

MGMT Expression and Resistance to TMZ

DNA repair and apoptosis are important chemoresistance mechanisms, especially when alkylating agents such as TMZ are involved.

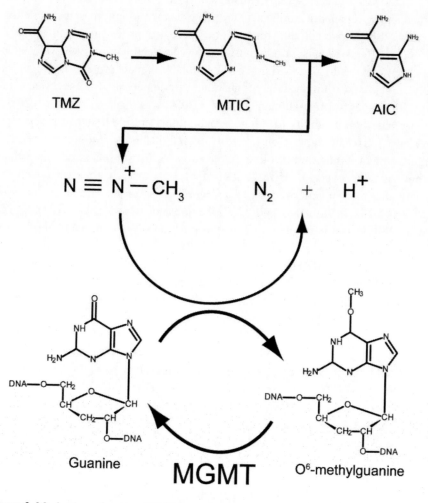

Figure 2. Mechanism of action of TMZ. TMZ is converted to 5-(3-methyltriazen-1-yl)imidazole-4-carboximide (MTIC) in water/blood with little or no enzymatic component. MTIC is broken down to methyldiazonium cation and 5-aminoimidazole-4-carboxamide (AIC). AIC is excreted via kidneys and methyldiazonium cations deliver methyl groups to DNA. Methyl groups are transferred to the 6th position oxygen atoms of guanines and O6-methylguanines are formed. O6-methylguanine mispairs with thymine instead of cytosine during DNA replication. The O6-methylguanine causes DNA break and apoptosis. MGMT removes methyl groups from O6-methylguanines to repair the genome. The expression of MGMT is epigenetically controlled. If the promoter region is methylated, the expression of MGMT is kept in low level.

Removal of alkyl groups, mismatch repair, base excision repair, and strand break repair are implicated in the resistance of gliomas to alkylating agents [28]. Above all, the removal of alkyl groups is suggested to have profound effects because a relationship between treatment and MGMT status has been observed [11, 29-31]. MGMT is a DNA repair protein that reverses alkylation at the O6 position of guanine to compensate for the effects of alkylating agents [32]. Human *MGMT* cDNA was isolated from a cDNA library based on its ability to rescue a methyltransferase-deficient *Escherichia coli* host [33]. The expression level of *MGMT* differs depending on species, organ, type of tumor, and cell line. In the early 1990s, subsets of cell lines that expressed low levels of *MGMT*, termed Mer- strains, were investigated to clarify the mechanism of decreased *MGMT* expression, and a correlation between DNA methylation and *MGMT* expression was revealed [34]. TMZ causes cell death by alkylation of the O6 position of guanine and subsequent disturbance of DNA replication; therefore, *MGMT* expression was implicated in resistance to TMZ chemotherapy. Indeed, *MGMT* expression and its contribution to resistance against TMZ have been reported in gliomas [35, 36]. Deletion, mutation, rearrangement, and mRNA instability of the *MGMT* gene are rare [37-41], and hypermethylation of the CpG island has been reported as the essential mechanism for *MGMT* silencing [29-31, 34, 37, 42-46]. Esteller et al. indicated that 40% of GBM cell lines, 50% of anaplastic astrocytoma cases, and 41% of GBM cases showed *MGMT* promoter methylation [37]. The incidence of *MGMT* promoter methylation in patients with GBM was 45% in the EORTC trial and the National Cancer Institute of Canada (NCSC) trial [11]. The MGMT protein level in tumor tissues can be evaluated by immunohistochemistry [47], and the activity of MGMT is measurable by an enzyme assay [48]. *MGMT* mRNA can be evaluated with reverse transcription-PCR (RT-PCR) [49] and real-time RT-PCR [50]. The methylation status of the *MGMT* gene has been assessed with methylation-specific PCR using bisulfite-modified DNA samples [45]. For diagnostic purposes, methylation-specific PCR is more advantageous than measurement of MGMT protein activity or mRNA levels because tissue contamination with non-neoplastic cells does not interfere with the detection of genomic methylation in tumor cells [30, 51]. To date, methylation-specific PCR is widely used for the evaluation of MGMT, although a standardized and validated method for the evaluation of MGMT status is required for the diagnosis and prognostication of gliomas. On the other hand, the clinical significance of *MGMT* promoter methylation status remains controversial [52, 53].

Chemoresistance Mechanisms Independent of MGMT

The enzymatic activity of MGMT is the most important mechanism underlying resistance to TMZ. However, other DNA repair and apoptosis processes exist, and other unknown mechanisms may also be present. The mismatch repair system is thought to be one mechanism of TMZ resistance [54-56]. Yip et al. reported mutations in the mismatch repair gene *MSH6* and microsatellite instability in patients with GBM after exposure to TMZ. These authors suggested that MSH6 inactivation could be involved in therapeutic resistance along with other unknown mechanisms [56]. Felsberg et al. reported reduced expression of MSH2, MSH6, and PMS2 protein in recurrent glioblastomas and suggested the existence of a novel chemoresistance mechanism facilitated by these proteins and independent of MGMT methylation [57]. The nucleotide excision repair system may also be involved in the TMZ resistance [58-62]. More than 80% of the DNA lesions methylated by TMZ are N-methylated bases that are recognized not by MGMT but rather by DNA glycosylases. Thus, resistance to TMZ may be due in part to robust base excision repair (BER) [58]. Knockdown of the BER enzyme DNA polymerase beta increased TMZ-induced cytotoxicity [59]. Some human tumor cells treated with TMZ showed increased expression of the chromatin-associated gene poly(ADP-ribose) polymerase-1 (*PARP-1*), which is involved in nucleotide excision repair [60]. PARP inhibitors have been shown to enhance sensitivity to TMZ [60-63].TMZ chemotherapy is expected not only to be a cytotoxic modality but also to sensitize tumor cells to radiation effects. TMZ actually enhances the radiosensitivity of tumor cells [64], and the strand break repair system is thought to interrupt this effect. Although TMZ can disrupt Rad51-induced repair [64], knockdown of the Rad54-related repair gene *DNA ligase IV* resulted in enhanced TMZ sensitivity in a human glioblastoma cell line [65]. The tumor suppressor p53 is a pleiotropic protein that plays an important role in DNA repair and apoptosis, and it functions via a mechanism distinct from that of MGMT. Wild-type p53 can reduce the cellular expression level of MGMT *in vitro* [66]. Conversely, in another report, p53 silencing reduced *MGMT* expression in murine astrocytic glioma cells [67]. Moreover, a p53 inhibitor enhanced the effects of TMZ in a mouse intracranial tumor implantation model, suggesting that p53 may induce the expression of *MGMT*, which in turn negatively regulates TMZ [68]. During treatment with chloroethylating agents, p53 protects against cell death;

however, this is not the case during treatment with methylating agents although both agents alkylate DNA [69]. The role of p53 during TMZ treatments has been described as favorable [66, 71, 72, 74], unfavorable [67, 68, 70], and variable depending on the type of cell [69, 73]. Collectively, the role of p53 is complicated and varies depending on cell type, *p53* allele (wild type or mutant), and type of agent.

Chemoresistance and Glioma Stem Cells

The concept of cancer stem cells is attracting increasing interest, and cancer stem cells may function as mediators of chemoresistance. Resistance to chemoradiotherapy may be due to the expansion of cancer stem cells, which can escape therapy-induced cell death. Cancer stem cells exhibit a multidrug-resistant phenotype by overexpressing drug transporters such as members of the adenosine triphosphate (ATP) binding cassette (ABC) superfamily and anti-apoptotic proteins such as B cell lymphoma/leukemia-2 (BCL-2) [75, 76]. CD133, CD15/SSEA-1, L1CAM, A2B5, and integrin α6 are some of the known surface markers that are used to enrich for glioma stem cells [77]. Additionally, glioma stem cells frequently express *MGMT* [78] and exhibit a multidrug resistant phenotype; thus, they may be more important therapeutic targets than the more highly differentiated tumor cells in the heterogeneous GBM population [77-79]. It has been reported that one of the ABC superfamily members, multidrug resistance 1 (MDR1), plays an important role in the chemoresistance of GBM independent of *MGMT* status [79]. Additionally, a single nucleotide polymorphism in the *MDR1* gene determines TMZ sensitivity [80]. A representative stem cell marker, CD133, was reported to be a candidate predictor of poor survival in patients treated with concomitant TMZ chemoradiotherapy [81, 82]. On the other hand, TMZ administration was also reported to decrease the number of glioma stem cells [83]. Conversely, treatment with BCNU increased the proportion of glioma stem cells in some cell lines [84].

Clinical Trials for GBM

Various phase II and III studies of malignant gliomas including GBM were performed and several studies are currently underway. Historically

important and recent phase II and III clinical studies of newly diagnosed GBM
[8, 9, 11, 17, 85-106] are shown in Table 1. TMZ and other alkylating agents
are elementary modalities involved in most of these trials. Importantly, TMZ
has become the standard of care for patients with GBM. On the other hand, an
overall survival longer than 2 years has not been shown in any clinical trials
except for a study of selected cases in which the patients had better
performance statuses [105]. Many clinical trials exploring treatments for
recurrent GBM, designated as salvage therapies, have also been performed.
Most of these therapies involve a combination of existing modalities and/or
alternative dose-dense schedules. Although efforts to utilize existing
modalities are important, breakthrough and innovative modalities are eagerly
anticipated for a complete cure of GBM.

**Table 1. Important and recent phase II and III clinical trials
for newly-diagnosed glioblastoma**

Reference	Year of publication	Remarks	Regimen	Patients (n)	Overall survival (months)
Levin et al. [8]	1990	NCOG	PCV + radiation	31	11.8
Weller et al. [9]	2003	NOA-01	ACNU + teniposide + radiation	154	17.3
Buckner et al. [85]	2006		cisplatin + BCNU + radiation	451	10.5
Colman et al. [86]	2006	RTOG9710	interferon beta + radiation	109	13.6
Westphal et al. [17]	2006		BCNU polymer wafers (Gliadel) + radiation	59	13.8
Brown et al. [87]	2008		erlotinib + TMZ + radiation	97	15.3
Stupp et al. [11]	2009	EORTC-NCIC	TMZ + radiation	287	14.6
Prados et al. [88]	2009		erlotinib + TMZ + radiation	65	19.3
Grossman et al. [89]	2009		Talampanel + TMZ + radiation	72	18.3
Beier et al. [90]	2009		pegylated liposomal doxorubicin + TMZ + radiation	63	17.6
Balducci et al. [91]	2010		TMZ + radiation	25	18
Mizumoto et al. [92]	2010		hyperfructionated proton radiation	20	21.6

Table 1. (Continued)

Reference	Year of publication	Remarks	Regimen	Patients (n)	Overall survival (months)
Jaeckle et al. [93]	2010	NCCTG	irinotecan + radiation	24	10.8
Jenkinson et al. [94]	2010		BCNU (intratumoral injection)	8	11.8
Peereboom et al. [95]	2010		erlotinib + TMZ + radiation	27	8.6
Li et al. [96]	2010		(125)I-mAb + TMZ + radiation	60	20.2
Hainsworth et al. [97]	2010		sorafenib + TMZ + radiation	47	12
Lai et al. [98]	2011		bevacizumab + TMZ + radiotherapy	70	19.6
Balducci et al. [99]	2011		TMZ + radiation (stereotactic)	36	28
Stummer et al. [100]	2011		fluorescence-guided resection + TMZ + radiation	122	16.3
Ogawa et al. [101]	2011		modified PCV + radiation + hyperbaric oxygenation	39	17.2
Butowski et al. [102]	2011		enzastaurin + TMZ + radiation	66	17.3
Ananda et al. [103]	2011		TMZ + pegylsted liposomal doxorubicin + radiation	40	13.4
Gállego Pérez-Larraya et al. [104]	2011	ANOCEF phase II	TMZ	70	5.8
Cho et al. [105]	2011		immunotherapy + TMZ + radiation	18	31.9
Ardon et al. [106]	2011	HGG-2006 phase I/II	immunotherapy + TMZ + radiation	77	18.3

Abbreviation; NCOG, the Northern California Oncology Group; NOA, Neuro-Oncology Working Group (of the German Cancer Society); RTOG, Radiation Therapy Oncology Group; EORTC, European Organization for the Research and Treatment of Cancer; NCIC, the National Cancer Institute of Canada Clinical Trials Group; NCCTG, the North Central Cancer Treatment Group; ANOCEF, Association des Neuro-Oncologuesd' Expression Française; HGG-2006, Immunotherapy for High Grade Glioma 2006 trial; PCV, procarbazine, CCNU, and vincristine.

Conclusion

Chemotherapy is an essential component in the multidisciplinary treatment of malignant gliomas. Alkylating agents such as TMZ and BCNU play major roles in current chemotherapy regimens. However, it remains controversial whether TMZ represents an improvement over conventional nitrosoureas [21, 107]. Nonetheless, regimens such as PCV-3 [8] and Stupp's regimen [10] will be important in postoperative adjuvant chemotherapy for the foreseeable future. Although the new alkylating agent TMZ has improved the prognosis of GBM and had an impact on the treatment of malignant gliomas, GBM remains an incurable disease. In order to attain a complete cure, new breakthroughs will be required. Treatment selection based on the molecular mechanisms of glioma pathogenesis and drug effects will become an integral part of personalized medicine; the role of *MGMT* methylation status as a predictive indicator of TMZ efficacy represents an illustrative example. In addition to translational approaches and improvements in drug delivery applications, an understanding of the molecular and cellular biology of gliomas, especially regarding chemoresistance and stem cell phenotype, will be required. The detailed molecular mechanisms of chemoresistance and the roles of related molecules including MGMT, mismatch repair enzymes, DNA excision repair enzymes, the ABC superfamily, and apoptosis-related factors will aid further innovation in the treatment of malignant gliomas.

Acknowledgement

This work was supported by a Grant-in-Aid for Young Scientists (B) 24590486 from the Ministry of Education, Culture, Sports, Science, and Technology of Japan.

References

[1]   Burton, EC; Prados, MD. Malignant gliomas. *Curr. Treat Options Oncol.*, 2000 1(5), 459-468.

[2]   Chamberlain, MC; Kormanik, PA. Practical guidelines for the treatment of malignant gliomas. *West J. Med.*, 1998 168(2), 114-120.

[3]   Lefranc, F; Sadeghi, N; Camby, I; Metens, T; Dewitte, O; Kiss, R. Present and potential future issues in glioblastoma treatment. *Expert. Rev. Anticancer Ther.*, 2006 6(5), 719-732.

[4]   Ammirati, M; Vick, N; Liao, YL; Ciric, I; Mikhael, M. Effect of the extent of surgical resection on survival and quality of life in patients with supratentorial glioblastomas and anaplastic astrocytomas. *Neurosurgery*, 1987 21(2), 201-206.

[5]   Stummer, W; Pichlmeier, U; Meinel, T; Wiestler, OD; Zanella, F; Reulen, HJ. Fluorescence-guided surgery with 5-aminolevulinic acid for resection of malignant glioma: a randomised controlled multicentre phase III trial. *Lancet Oncol.*, 2006 7(5), 392-401.

[6]   Walker, MD; Alexander, E Jr; Hunt, WE; MacCarty, CS; Mahaley, MS Jr; Mealey, J Jr; et al. Evaluation of BCNU and/or radiotherapy in the treatment of anaplastic gliomas. A cooperative clinical trial. *J. Neuro surg.*, 1978 49(3), 333-343.

[7]   Walker, MD; Strike, TA; Sheline, GE. An analysis of dose-effect relationship in the radiotherapy of malignant gliomas. *Int. J. Radiat. Oncol. Biol. Phys.*, 1979 5(10), 1725-1731.

[8]   Levin, VA; Silver, P; Hannigan, J; Wara, WM; Gutin, PH; Davis, RL; et al. Superiority of post-radiotherapy adjuvant chemotherapy with CCNU, procarbazine, and vincristine (PCV) over BCNU for anaplastic gliomas: NCOG 6G61 final report. *J. Rad. Onc. Biol. Phys.*, 1990 18(2), 321-324.

[9]   Weller, M; Muller, B; Koch, R; Bamberg, M; Krauseneck, P; Neuro-Oncology Working Group of the German Cancer Society. Neuro-Oncology Working Group 01 trial of nimustine plus teniposide versus nimustine plus cytarabine chemotherapy in addition to involved-field radiotherapy in the first-line treatment of malignant gliomas. *J. Clin. Oncol.*, 2003 21(17), 3276-3284.

[10] Stupp, R; Mason, WP; van den Bent, MJ; Weller, M; Fisher, B; Taphoorn, MJ; et al. Radiotherapy plus concomitant and adjuvant temozolomide for glioblastoma. *N. Engl. J. Med.*, 2005 352(10), 987-996.

[11] Stupp, R; Hegi, ME; Mason, WP; van den Bent, MJ; Taphoorn, MJ; Janzer, RC; et al. Effects of radiotherapy with concomitant and adjuvant temozolomide versus radiotherapy alone on survival in glioblastoma in a randomised phase III study: 5-year analysis of the EORTC-NCIC trial. *Lancet Oncol.*, 2009 10(5), 459-466.

[12] Khasraw, M; Lassman, AB. Advances in the treatment of malignant gliomas. *Curr. Oncol. Rep.*, 2010 12(1), 26-33.

[13] Villano, JL; Seery, TE; Bressler, LR. Temozolomide in malignant gliomas: current use and future targets. *Cancer Chemother. Pharmacol.*, 2009 64(4), 647-655.

[14] Gonzaga, PE; Potter, PM; Niu, TQ; Yu, D; Ludlum, DB; Rafferty, JA; et al. Identification of the cross-link between human O6-methylguanine-DNA methyltransferase and chloroethylnitrosourea-treated DNA. *Cancer Res.*, 1992 52(21), 6052-6058.

[15] Chabner, BA; Amrein, PC; Druker, BJ; Michaelson, MD; Mitsidiades, CS; Goss, PE; et al. Antineoplastic agents. In Brunton, LL (eds.), Goodman and Gilman's the Pharmacological Basis of Therapeutics (11th ed., 1315-1335). New York, NY: McGraw-Hill: 2006.

[16] Shapiro, WR; Green, SB; Burger, PC; Selker, RG; VanGilder, JC; Robertson, JT; et al. A randomized comparison of intra-arterial versus intravenous BCNU, with or without intravenous 5-fluorouracil, for newly diagnosed patients with malignant glioma. *J. Neuro surg.*, 1992 76(5), 772-781.

[17] Westphal, M; Ram, Z; Riddle, V; Hilt, D; Bortey, E. (Executive Committee of the Gliadel Study Group). Gliadel wafer in initial surgery for malignant glioma: long-term follow-up of a multicenter controlled trial. *Acta Neurochir.* (Wien), 2006 148(3), 269-275.

[18] Levin, VA; Silver, P; Hannigan, J; Wara, WM; Gutin, PH; Davis, RL; et al. Superiority of post-radiotherapy adjuvant chemotherapy with CCNU, procarbazine, and vincristine (PCV) over BCNU for anaplastic gliomas: NCOG 6G61 final report. *Int. J. Radiat. Oncol. Biol. Phys.*, 1990 18(2), 321-324.

[19] Cairncross, JG; Ueki, K; Zlatescu, MC; Lisle, DK; Finkelstein, DM; Hammond, RR; et al. Specific genetic predictors of chemotherapeutic response and survival in patients with anaplastic oligodendrogliomas. *J. Natl. Cancer Inst.*, 1998 90(19), 1473-1479.

[20] Smith, JS; Perry, A; Borell, TJ; Lee, HK; O'Fallon, J; Hosek, SM; et al. Alterations of chromosome arms 1p and 19q as predictors of survival in oligodendrogliomas, astrocytomas, and mixed oligoastrocytomas. *J. Clin. Oncol.*, 2000 18(3), 636-645.

[21] Linz, U. Chemotherapy for glioblastoma: is costly better? *Cancer*, 2008 113(10), 2617-2622.

[22] Stevens, MF; Hickman, JA; Stone, R; Gibson, NW; Baig, GU; Lunt, E; et al. Antitumor imidazotetrazines. 1. Synthesis and chemistry of 8-carbamoyl-3-(2-chloroethyl)imidazo[5,1-d]-1,2,3,5-tetrazin-4(3 H)-one,

a novel broad-spectrum antitumor agent. *J. Med. Chem.*, 1984 27(2), 196-201.

[23] Newlands, ES; Blackledge, G; Slack, JA; Goddard, C; Brindley, CJ; Holden, L; et al. Phase I clinical trial of mitozolomide. *Cancer Treat Rep.*, 1985 69(7-8), 801-805.

[24] Stevens, MF; Hickman, JA; Langdon, SP; Chubb, D; Vickers, L; Stone, R; et al. Antitumor activity and pharmacokinetics in mice of 8-carbamoyl-3-methyl-imidazo[5,1-d]-1,2,3,5-tetrazin-4(3H)-one (CCRG 81045; MandB 39831), a novel drug with potential as an alternative to dacarbazine. *Cancer Res.*, 1987 47(22), 5846-5852.

[25] Newlands, ES; Blackledge, GR; Slack, JA; Rustin, GJ; Smith, DB; Stuart, NS; et al. Phase I trial of temozolomide (CCRG 81045: MandB 39831: NSC 362856). *Br. J. Cancer*, 1992 65(2), 287-291.

[26] Clark, AS; Deans, B; Stevens, MF; Tisdale, MJ; Wheelhouse, RT; Denny, BJ; et al. Antitumor imidazotetrazines. 32. Synthesis of novel imidazotetrazinones and related bicyclic heterocycles to probe the mode of action of the antitumor drug temozolomide. *J. Med. Chem.*, 1995 38(9), 1493-1504.

[27] Denny, BJ; Wheelhouse, RT; Stevens, MF; Tsang, LL; Slack, JA. NMR and molecular modeling investigation of the mechanism of activation of the antitumor drug temozolomide and its interaction with DNA. *Biochemistry*, 1994 33(31), 9045-9051.

[28] Frosina, G. DNA repair and resistance of gliomas to chemotherapy and radiotherapy. *Mol. Cancer Res.*, 2009 7(7), 989-999.

[29] Estellar, M; Garcia-Foncillas, J; Andion, E; Goodman, SN; Hidalgo, OF; Vanaclocha, V; et al. Inactivation of the DNA-repair gene MGMT and the clinical response of gliomas to alkylating agents. *N. Engl. J. Med.*, 2000 343(19), 1350-1354.

[30] Hegi, ME; Liu, L; Herman, JG; Stupp, R; Wick, W; Weller, M; et al. Correlation of O6-methylguanine methyltransferase (MGMT) promoter methylation with clinical outcomes in glioblastoma and clinical strategies to modulate MGMT activity. *J. Clin. Oncol.*, 2008 26(25), 4189-4199.

[31] Hegi, ME; Diserens, AC; Gorlia, T; Hamou, M. F; de Tribolet, N; Weller, M; et al. MGMT gene silencing and benefit from temozolomide in glioblastoma. *N. Engl. J. Med.*, 2005 352(10), 997-1003.

[32] Dolan, ME; Moschel, RC; Pegg, AE. Depletion of mammalian O6-alkylguanine-DNA alkyltransferase activity by O6-benzylguanine provides a means to evaluate the role of this protein in protection against

carcinogenic and therapeutic alkylating agents. *Proc. Natl. Acad. Sci. USA*, 1990 87(14), 5368-5372.

[33]   Tano, K; Shiota, S; Collier J; Foote R. S; Mitra, S. (1990). Isolation and structural characterization of a cDNA clone encoding the human DNA repair protein for O6-alkylguanine. *Proc. Natl. Acad. Sci. USA*, 87, 686-690.

[34]   Wang, Y; Kato, T; Ayaki, H; Ishizaki, K; Tano, K; Mitra, S; et al. Correlation between DNA methylation and expression of O6-methylguanine-DNA methyltransferase gene in cultured human tumor cells. *Mutat. Res.*, 1992 273(2), 221-230.

[35]   Preuss, I; Eberhagen, I; Haas, S; Eibl, RH; Kaufmann, M; von Minckwitz, G; Kaina B. O6-methylguanine-DNA methyltransferase activity in breast and brain tumors. *Int. J. Cancer*, 1995 61(3), 321-326.

[36]   Bobola, MS; Tseng SH; Blank A; Berger MS; Silber JR. Role of O6-methylguanine-DNA methyltransferase in resistance of human brain tumor cell lines to the clinically relevant methylating agents temozolomide and streptozotocin. *Clin. Cancer Res.*, 1996 2(4), 735-741.

[37]   Esteller, M; Hamilton, SR; Burger, PC; Baylin, SB; Herman, JG. Inactivation of the DNA repair gene O6-methylguanine-DNA methyltransferase by promoter hypermethylation is a common event in primary human neoplasia. *Cancer Res.*, 1999 59(4), 793-797.

[38]   Day, RS 3rd; Ziolkowski, CH; Scudiero, DA; Meyer, SA; Lubiniecki, AS; Girardi, AJ; et al. Defective repair of alkylated DNA by human tumor and SV40-transformed human cell strains. *Nature*, 1980 288(5792), 724-727.

[39]   Fornace, AJ Jr; Papathanasiou, MA; Hollander, MC; Yarosh, DB. Expression of the O6-methylguanine DNA methyltransferase gene MGMT in MER+ and MER- human tumor cells. *Cancer Res.*, 1990 50(24), 7908-7911.

[40]   Pieper, RO; Futscher, BW; Dong, Q; Ellis, TM; Erickson, LC. Comparison of O6-methylguanine-DNA methyltransferase gene (MGMT) mRNA levels in MER+ and MER- human tumor cell lines containing the MGMT gene by the polymerase chain reaction technique. *Cancer Commun.*, 1990 2(1), 13-20.

[41]   Kroes, RA; Erickson, LC. The role of mRNA stability and transcription in O6-methylguanine-DNA methyltransferase (MGMT) expression in Mer- human tumor cell lines. *Carcinogenesis*, 1995 16(9), 2255-2257.

[42] Costello, JF; Futscher, BW; Tano, K; Graunke, DM; Pieper, RO. Graded
      methylation in the promoter and in the body of the O6-methylguanine-
      DNA methyltransferase gene correlates with MGMT expression in
      human glioma cells. *Cancer Res.*, 1994 269(25), 17228-17237.
[43] Qian, XC; Brent, TP. Methylation hot spots in the 5'-flanking region
      denote silencing of the O6-Methylguanine-DNA methyltransferase gene.
      Cancer Res., 1997 57(17), 3672-3677.
[44] Watts, GS; Pieper, RO; Costello, JF; Peng, Y-M; Dalton, WS; Futscher,
      BW. Methylation of discrete regions of the O6-Methylguanine DNA
      methyltransferase (MGMT) CpG island is associated with
      heterochromatinization of the MGMT transcription start site and
      silencing of the gene. *Mol. Cell Biol.*, 1997 17(9), 5612-5619.
[45] Paz, MF; Yaya-Tur, R; Rojas-Marcos, I; Reynes, G; Pollan, M; Aguirre-
      Cruz, L; et al. CpG island hypermethylation of the DNA repair enzyme
      methyltransferase predicts response to temozolomide in primary
      gliomas. *Clin. Cancer Res.*, 2004 10(15), 4933-4938.
[46] Hegi, ME; Diserens, AC; Godard, S; Dietrich, PY; Regli, L; Ostermann,
      S; et al. Clinical trial substantiates the predictive value of O-6-
      methylguanine-DNA methyltransferase promoter methylation in
      glioblastoma patients treated with temozolomide. *Clin. Cancer Res.*,
      2004 10(6), 1871-1874.
[47] Sasai, K; Nodagashira, M; Nishihara, H; Aoyanagi, E; Wang, L; Katoh,
      M; et al. Careful Exclusion of Non-neoplastic Brain Components is
      Required for an Appropriate Evaluation of O6-methylguanine-DNA
      methyltransferase status in glioma: relationship between
      immunohistochemistry and methylation analysis. *Am. J. Surg. Pathol.*,
      2008 32(8), 1220-1227.
[48] Spiro, TP; Gerson, SL; Liu, L; Majka, S; Haaga, J; Hoppel, CL; et al.
      O6-benzylguanine: a clinical trial establishing the biochemical
      modulatory dose in tumor tissue for alkyltransferase-directed DNA
      repair. *Cancer Res.*, 1999 59(10), 2402-2410.
[49] Mineura, K; Yanagisawa, T; Watanabe, K; Kowada, M; Yasui, N.
      Human brain tumor O(6)-methylguanine-DNA methyltransferase
      mRNA and its significance as an indicator of selective chloroethyl
      nitrosourea chemotherapy. *Int. J. Cancer*, 1996 69(5), 420-425.
[50] Tanaka, S; Kobayashi, I; Utsuki, S; Oka, H; Fujii, K; Watanabe, T; et al.
      O6-methylguanine-DNA methyltranspherase gene expression in gliomas
      by means of real-time quantitative RT-PCR and clinical response to
      nitrosoureas. *Int. J. Cancer*, 2003 103(1), 67-72.

[51] Rodriguez, FJ; Thibodeau, SN; Jenkins, RB; Schowalter, KV; Caron, BL; O'neill, BP; et al. MGMT immunohistochemical expression and promoter methylation in human glioblastoma. *Appl. Immunohistochem. Mol. Morphol.*, 2008 16(1), 59-65.

[52] Weller, M. Novel diagnostic and therapeutic approaches to malignant glioma. Swiss Med Wkly, 2011 141, w13210 (doi:10.4414/ smw.2011.13210).

[53] Jha, P; Suri, V; Jain, A; Sharma, MC; Pathak, P; Jha, P; et al. O6-methylguanine DNA methyltransferase gene promoter methylation status in gliomas and its correlation with other molecular alterations: first Indian report with review of challenges for use in customized treatment. *Neurosurgery*, 2010 67(6), 1681-1691.

[54] Friedman, HS; Johnson, SP; Dong, Q; Schold, SC; Rasheed, BK; Bigner, SH; et al. Methylator resistance mediated by mismatch repair deficiency in a glioblastoma multiforme xenograft. *Cancer Res.*, 1997 57(14), 2933-2936.

[55] Liu, L; Markowitz, S; Gerson, SL. Mismatch repair mutations override alkyltransferase in conferring resistance to temozolomide but not to 1,3-bis(2-chloroethyl)nitrosourea. *Cancer Res.*, 1996 56(23), 5375-5379.

[56] Yip, S; Miao, J; Cahill, DP; Iafrate, AJ; Aldape, K; Nutt, CL; et al. MSH6 mutations arise in glioblastomas during temozolomide therapy and mediate temozolomide resistance. *Clin. Cancer Res.*, 2009 15(14), 4622-4629.

[57] Felsberg, J; Thon, N; Eigenbrod, S; Hentschel, B; Sabel, MC; Westphal, M; et al. Promoter methylation and expression of MGMT and the DNA mismatch repair genes MLH1, MSH2, MSH6 and PMS2 in paired primary and recurrent glioblastomas. *Int. J. Cancer*, 2011 129(3), 659-670.

[58] Trivedi, RN; Almeida, KH; Fornsaglio, JL; Schamus, S; Sobol, RW. The role of base excision repair in the sensitivity and resistance to temozolomide-mediated cell death. *Cancer Res.*, 2005 65(14), 6394-6400.

[59] Liu, L; Taverna, P; Whitacre, CM; Chatterjee, S; Gerson, SL. Pharmacologic disruption of base excision repair sensitizes mismatch repair-deficient and -proficient colon cancer cells to methylating agents. *Clin. Cancer Res.*, 1999 5(10), 2908-2917.

[60] Tentori, L; Portarena, I; Torino, F; Scerrati, M; Navarra, P; Graziani, G. Poly(ADP-ribose) polymerase inhibitor increases growth inhibition and

reduces G(2)/M cell accumulation induced by temozolomide in malignant glioma cells. *Glia,* 2002 40(1), 44-54.

[61] Curtin, NJ; Wang, LZ; Yiakouvaki, A; Kyle, S; Arris, CA; Canan-Koch, S; et al. Novel poly(ADP-ribose) polymerase-1 inhibitor, AG14361, restores sensitivity to temozolomide in mismatch repair-deficient cells. *Clin. Cancer Res.,* 2004 10(3), 881-889.

[62] Dungey, FA; Löser, DA; Chalmers, AJ. Replication-dependent radiosensitization of human glioma cells by inhibition of poly(ADP-Ribose) polymerase: mechanisms and therapeutic potential. *Int. J. Radiat. Oncol. Biol. Phys.,* 2008 72(4), 1188-1197.

[63] Tentori, L; Leonetti, C; Scarsella, M; d'Amati, G; Portarena, I; Zupi, G; et al. Combined treatment with temozolomide and poly(ADP-ribose) polymerase inhibitor enhances survival of mice bearing hematologic malignancy at the central nervous system site. *Blood,* 2002 99(6), 2241-2224.

[64] Kil, WJ; Cerna, D; Burgan, WE; Beam, K; Carter, D; Steeg, PS; et al. In vitro and in vivo radiosensitization induced by the DNA methylating agent temozolomide. *Clin. Cancer Res.,* 2008 14(3), 931-938.

[65] Kondo, N; Takahashi, A; Mori, E; Ohnishi, K; McKinnon, PJ; Sakaki, T. DNA ligase IV as a new molecular target for temozolomide. *Biochem. Biophys. Res. Commun.,* 2009 387(4), 656-660.

[66] Harris, L. C; Remack, JS; Houghton, PJ; Brent, TP. Wild-type p53 suppresses transcription of the human O6-methylguanine-DNA methyltransferase gene. *Cancer Res.,* 1996 56(9), 2029-2032.

[67] Blough, MD; Zlatescu, MC; Cairncross, JG. O6-methylguanine-DNA methyltransferase regulation by p53 in astrocytic cells. *Cancer Res.,* 2007 67(2), 580-584.

[68] Dinca, EB; Lu, KV; Sarkaria, JN; Pieper, RO; Prados, MD; Haas-Kogan, DA; et al. p53 Small-molecule inhibitor enhances temozolomide cytotoxic activity against intracranial glioblastoma xenografts. *Cancer Res.,* 2008 68(24), 10034-10039.

[69] Batista, LF; Roos, WP; Christmann, M; Menck, CF; Kaina, B. Differential sensitivity of malignant glioma cells to methylating and chloroethylating anticancer drugs: p53 determines the switch by regulating xpc, ddb2, and DNA double-strand breaks. *Cancer Res.,* 2007 67(24), 11886-11895.

[70] Li, S; Zhang, W; Chen, B; Jiang, T; Wang, Z. Prognostic and predictive value of p53 in low MGMT expressing glioblastoma treated with

surgery, radiation and adjuvant temozolomide chemotherapy. *Neurol. Res.*, 2010 32(7), 690-694.

[71] Bocangel, D; Sengupta, S; Mitra, S; Bhakat, KK. p53-Mediated down-regulation of the human DNA repair gene O6-methylguanine-DNA methyltransferase (MGMT) via interaction with Sp1 transcription factor. *Anticancer Res.*, 2009 29(10), 3741-3750.

[72] Bobustuc, GC; Baker, CH; Limaye, A; Jenkins, WD; Pearl, G; Avgeropoulos, NG; et al. Levetiracetam enhances p53-mediated MGMT inhibition and sensitizes glioblastoma cells to temozolomide. *Neuro Oncol.*, 2010 12(9), 917-927.

[73] Blough, MD; Beauchamp, DC; Westgate, MR; Kelly, JJ; Cairncross, JG. Effect of aberrant p53 function on temozolomide sensitivity of glioma cell lines and brain tumor initiating cells from glioblastoma. *J. Neuro oncol.*, 2011 102(1), 1-7.

[74] Sato, A; Sunayama, J; Matsuda, K; Seino, S; Suzuki, K; Watanabe, E; et al. MEK-ERK signaling dictates DNA-repair gene MGMT expression and temozolomide resistance of stem-like glioblastoma cells via the MDM2-p53 axis. *Stem. Cells*, 2011 29 (12), 1942-1951.

[75] Singh, SK; Clarke, ID; Hide, T; Dirks, PB. Cancer stem cells in nervous system tumors. *Oncogene*, 2004 23(43), 7267-7273.

[76] Lu, C; Shervington, A. Chemoresistance in gliomas. Mol Cell Biochem, 2008 312(1-2), 71-80.

[77] Venere, M; Fine, HA; Dirks, PB; Rich, JN. Cancer stem cells in gliomas: identifying and understanding the apex cell in cancer's hierarchy. *Glia*, 2011 59(8), 1148-1154.

[78] Beier, D; Schulz, JB; Beier, CP. Chemoresistance of glioblastoma cancer stem cells--much more complex than expected. *Mol. Cancer*, 2011 10, 128 (doi:10.1186/1476-4598-10-128)

[79] Nakai, E; Park, K; Yawata, T; Chihara, T; Kumazawa, A; Nakabayashi, H; et al. Enhanced MDR1 expression and chemoresistance of cancer stem cells derived from glioblastoma. *Cancer Invest.*, 2009 27(9), 901-908.

[80] Schaich, M; Kestel, L; Pfirrmann, M; Robel, K; Illmer, T; Kramer, M; et al. A MDR1 (ABCB1) gene single nucleotide polymorphism predicts outcome of temozolomide treatment in glioblastoma patients. *Ann. Oncol.*, 2009 20(1), 175-181.

[81] Murat, A; Migliavacca, E; Gorlia, T; Lambiv, WL; Shay, T; Hamou, MF; et al. Stem cell-related "self-renewal" signature and high epidermal growth factor receptor expression associated with resistance to

concomitant chemoradiotherapy in glioblastoma. *J. Clin. Oncol.*, 2008 26(18), 3015-3024.

[82] Pallini, R; Ricci-Vitiani, L; Banna, GL; Signore, M; Lombardi, D; Todaro, M; et al. Cancer stem cell analysis and clinical outcome in patients with glioblastoma multiforme. *Clin. Cancer Res.*, 2008 14(24), 8205-8212.

[83] Beier, D; Röhrl, S; Pillai, DR; Schwarz, S; Kunz-Schughart, LA; Leukel, P; et al. Temozolomide preferentially depletes cancer stem cells in glioblastoma. *Cancer Res.*, 2008 68(14), 5706-5715.

[84] Kang, MK; Kang, SK. Tumorigenesis of chemotherapeutic drug-resistant cancer stem-like cells in brain glioma. *Stem. Cells Dev.*, 2007 16(5), 837-847.

[85] Buckner, JC; Ballman, KV; Michalak, JC; Burton; GV, Cascino; TL, Schomberg, PJ; et al. North Central Cancer Treatment Group 93-72-52; Southwest Oncology Group 9503 Trials. Phase III trial of carmustine and cisplatin compared with carmustine alone and standard radiation therapy or accelerated radiation therapy in patients with glioblastoma multiforme: North Central Cancer Treatment Group 93-72-52 and Southwest Oncology Group 9503 Trials. *J. Clin. Oncol.*, 2006 24(24), 3871-3879.

[86] Colman, H; Berkey, BA; Maor, MH; Groves, MD; Schultz, CJ; Vermeulen, S; et al. Radiation Therapy Oncology Group. Phase II Radiation Therapy Oncology Group trial of conventional radiation therapy followed by treatment with recombinant interferon-beta for supratentorial glioblastoma: results of RTOG 9710. *Int. J. Radiat. Oncol. Biol. Phys.*, 2006 66(3), 818-824.

[87] Brown, PD, Krishnan, S, Sarkaria, JN, Wu, W, Jaeckle, KA, Uhm, JH, et al. North Central Cancer Treatment Group Study N0177. Phase I/II trial of erlotinib and temozolomide with radiation therapy in the treatment of newly diagnosed glioblastoma multiforme: North Central Cancer Treatment Group Study N0177. *J. Clin. Oncol.*, 2008 26(34), 5603-5609.

[88] Prados, MD; Chang, SM; Butowski, N; DeBoer, R; Parvataneni R; Carliner, H; et al. Phase II study of erlotinib plus temozolomide during and after radiation therapy in patients with newly diagnosed glioblastoma multiforme or gliosarcoma. *J. Clin. Oncol.*, 2009 27(4), 579-584.

[89] Grossman, SA; Ye, X; Chamberlain, M; Mikkelsen, T; Batchelor, T; Desideri, S; et al. Talampanel with standard radiation and temozolomide

in patients with newly diagnosed glioblastoma: a multicenter phase II trial. *J. Clin. Oncol.*, 2009 27(25), 4155-4161.

[90] Beier, CP; Schmid, C; Gorlia, T; Kleinletzenberger, C; Beier, D; Grauer, O; et al. RNOP-09: pegylated liposomal doxorubicine and prolonged temozolomide in addition to radiotherapy in newly diagnosed glioblastoma--a phase II study. *BMC Cancer*, 2009 9, 308 (doi:10.1186/1471-2407-9-308).

[91] Balducci, M; D'Agostino, GR; Manfrida, S; De Renzi, F; Colicchio, G; Apicella, G; et al. Radiotherapy and concomitant temozolomide during the first and last weeks in high grade gliomas: long-term analysis of a phase II study. *J. Neuro oncol.*, 2010 97(1), 95-100.

[92] Mizumoto, M; Tsuboi, K; Igaki, H; Yamamoto, T; Takano, S; Oshiro, Y; et al. Phase I/II trial of hyperfractionated concomitant boost proton radiotherapy for supratentorial glioblastoma multiforme. *Int. J. Radiat. Oncol. Biol. Phys.*, 2010 77(1), 98-105.

[93] Jaeckle, KA; Ballman, KV; Giannini, C; Schomberg, PJ; Ames, MM; Reid, JM; et al. Phase II NCCTG trial of RT + irinotecan and adjuvant BCNU plus irinotecan for newly diagnosed GBM. *J. Neuro oncol.*, 2010 99(1), 73-80.

[94] Jenkinson, MD; Smith, TS; Haylock, B; Husband, D; Shenoy, A; Vinjamuri, S; et al. Phase II trial of intratumoral BCNU injection and radiotherapy on untreated adult malignant glioma. *J. Neuro oncol.*, 2010 99(1), 103-113.

[95] Peereboom, DM; Shepard, DR; Ahluwalia, MS; Brewer, CJ; Agarwal, N; Stevens, GH; et al. Phase II trial of erlotinib with temozolomide and radiation in patients with newly diagnosed glioblastoma multiforme. *J. Neuro oncol.*, 2010 98(1), 93-99.

[96] Li, L; Quang, TS; Gracely, EJ; Kim, JH; Emrich, JG; Yaeger, TE; et al. A Phase II study of anti-epidermal growth factor receptor radioimmunotherapy in the treatment of glioblastoma multiforme. *J. Neuro surg.*, 2010 113(2), 192-198.

[97] Hainsworth, JD; Ervin, T; Friedman, E; Priego, V; Murphy, PB; Clark, BL; et al. Concurrent radiotherapy and temozolomide followed by temozolomide and sorafenib in the first-line treatment of patients with glioblastoma multiforme. *Cancer*, 2010 116(15), 3663-3669.

[98] Lai, A, Tran, A; Nghiemphu, PL; Pope, WB; Solis, OE; Selch, M; Filka, E; et al. Phase II study of bevacizumab plus temozolomide during and after radiation therapy for patients with newly diagnosed glioblastoma multiforme. *J. Clin. Oncol.*, 2011 29(2), 142-148.

[99] Balducci, M; Apicella, G; Manfrida, S; Mangiola, A; Fiorentino, A; Azario, L; et al. Single-arm phase II study of conformal radiation therapy and temozolomide plus fractionated stereotactic conformal boost in high-grade gliomas: final report. *Strahlenther Onkol.*, 2010 186(10), 558-564.

[100] Stummer, W; Nestler, U; Stockhammer, F; Krex, D; Kern, BC; Mehdorn, HM; et al. Favorable outcome in the elderly cohort treated by concomitant temozolomide radiochemotherapy in a multicentric phase II safety study of 5-ALA. *J. Neuro oncol.*, 2011 103(2), 361-370.

[101] Ogawa, K; Ishiuchi, S; Inoue, O; Yoshii, Y; Saito, A; Watanabe, T; et al. Phase II trial of radiotherapy after hyperbaric oxygenation with multiagent chemotherapy (procarbazine, nimustine, and vincristine) for high-grade gliomas: long-term results. *Int. J. Radiat. Oncol. Biol. Phys.*, 2012 82(2), 732-738.

[102] Butowski, N; Chang, SM; Lamborn, KR; Polley, MY; Pieper, R; Costello, JF; et al. Phase II and pharmacogenomics study of enzastaurin plus temozolomide during and following radiation therapy in patients with newly diagnosed glioblastoma multiforme and gliosarcoma. *Neuro Oncol.*, 2011 13(12), 1331-1338.

[103] Ananda, S; Nowak, AK; Cher, L; Dowling, A; Brown, C; Simes, J; et al. Cooperative Trials Group for Neuro-Oncology (COGNO). Phase 2 trial of temozolomide and pegylated liposomal doxorubicin in the treatment of patients with glioblastoma multiforme following concurrent radiotherapy and chemotherapy. *J. Clin. Neuro sci.*, 2011 18(11), 1444-1448.

[104] Gállego Pérez-Larraya, J; Ducray, F; Chinot, O; Catry-Thomas, I; Taillandier, L; Guillamo, JS; et al. Temozolomide in elderly patients with newly diagnosed glioblastoma and poor performance status: an ANOCEF phase II trial. *J. Clin. Oncol.*, 2011 29(22), 3050-3055.

[105] Cho, DY; Yang, WK; Lee, HC; Hsu, DM; Lin, HL; Lin, SZ; et al. Adjuvant immunotherapy with whole-cell lysate dendritic cells vaccine for glioblastoma multiforme: a phase II clinical trial. *World Neuro surg.*, 2012 77(5-6), 736-744.

[106] Ardon, H; Van Gool, SW; Verschuere, T; Maes, W; Fieuws, S; Sciot, R; et al. Integration of autologous dendritic cell-based immunotherapy in the standard of care treatment for patients with newly diagnosed glioblastoma: results of the HGG-2006 phase I/II trial. *Cancer Immunol. Immunother.*, 2012 61(11), 2033-2044.

[107] Wick, W; Hartmann, C; Engel, C; Stoffels, M; Felsberg, J; Stockhammer, F; et al. NOA-04 randomized phase III trial of sequential radiochemotherapy of anaplastic glioma with procarbazine, lomustine, and vincristine or temozolomide. *J. Clin. Oncol.*, 2009 27(35), 5874-5880.

Index

D

H

N

O

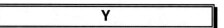

Y